HOW TO TAKE CARE OF YOURSELF FOR SUCCESS

¿What will you do know that you benefits discover the supplementation of medical plants and for high performance?

Valentín López

HOW TO TAKE CARE OF YOURSELF FOR SUCCESS

¿What will you do know that you benefits discover the supplementation of medical plants and for high performance?

Valentín López

ISBN: 9781717897374

AMAZON BESTSELLER #1

Genre: Personal Health & Beauty & Fitness

4th EDITION

First Edition: June 2018

Canary Islands Spain

You can contact us at:

clientes@valentinlopez.org

If you think we have given you value and want to contribute to our
causes, you can do so at the following link:

Contributions and retributions:

paypal.me/lopezvalentin

CONTENTS

Those who call you crazy are those
who have not had the courage to fight for their dreams.
But you know what?,
They are your limitations, not yours.

Valentín López

WHAT DO THEY SAY ABOUT VALENTÍN LÓPEZ AND *HOW TO TAKE CARE OF YOUR-SELF FOR SUCCESS?*

PROLOGUE OF ANA OLIVA

"If Valentín has put his time to write this book, read it deserves my full attention. Health and personal welfare concerns us all, a practical, simple and well documented book. Different and original, *How to take care of yourself for success* gives clear and to the point of the various principles that can help us guidelines at all times, I'm so glad I read".

"Valentín's present and future. It is always excited and fully committed to creating projects and this would not be the exception. A young man with determination does not wait for opportunities to reach their life simply out to look for them and as in this case, creates. Natas has qualities communicator, knows how to inspire people and how to connect. Knowing you and knowing how to think, *How to take care of yourself for success* it is the beginning of many other projects that I follow closely. "

"Good luck and happy way to our goals!, a hug".

Ana Oliva,
Journalist, Biographer, Coach for authors, Editorial
Digital Marketing, Author of more than 7 books, including:
"Antonio Banderas, a Life Film"
"Traders Success "or" My First Million"
anaoliva.com
Spain

"Success is a very personal thing for sure, but I agree with my friend Valentín López attitude is paramount to achieve, as well as skills and knowledge quality. No doubt this is a great book full of good information to be applied in our daily lives ".

"Health is our engine, take care and drive your life".

Abraham Viera,
Coach Team Viera and Physical Trainer
Multichampion National Bodybuilding
Spain

"Since I met Valentín López, I could see a great man, persevering, prosperous, full of abundance, love and blessing to give to others. Thanks to him I have learned to have more energy, encourage others to pursue their dreams, stay with the positive and spiritual well being grateful. I am sure that this book his work will be of great blessing and a tremendous advantage for those who have the good fortune to read it".

"Grateful for your great contribution to society because friend you help us continue to expand the purpose for which we are in life; to serve".

Dilu Pereda,
Speaker expert in Personal Image,
Marketing and Business
Peru

"Success demands more of our blood and sweat than ever, only those who recognize this truth and adjust your lifestyle to a healthier one, they are those who live to enjoy his glory days with the privilege of full health. Meet the nutrients both Valentín and other achievers will produce results, increasing productivity and responsiveness to stress, both essential to achieve and maintain the win".

Karina Carlos,
Lawyer, Life Coach and Speaker
Podcaster
Mexico

"I think in life there is nothing more noble and praiseworthy to help, and that's what characterizes Valentín López. Always projecting ideas to bene fi t others. *How to take care of yourself for success* it is a wonderful work, easy to read and accessible to all, which gives us tools to our well-being and a better quality of life".

Javier López,
Journalist, Radio Host
Argentina

"After reading the book Valentín López, I completely sure it will be a solid foundation to help the welfare of the people".

Muhammad Salah,
Doctor and Pharmacist
Egypt

"Valentín López is undoubtedly one of the most prepared and talented people I've ever met. His hunger to learn every day and to inspire others is really admirable. As I travel around the world (over 70 countries already), many know Valentín and tell me their messages on social networks have impacted many their lives. I'm super proud of his friendship, since we met in person we speak daily. Congratulations on this great project".

"This world would be much better with more people like Valentín".

Carlos Concheso,
Entrepreneur
USA

"I admire all those people who daily struggle for their dreams and help others do so. Valentín is one of them, which help for a common good, really must know, people like him are most needed in this world. As industry professional I think a very full, explicit, simple to understand and recommended for all public book. Thanks friend for approaching this beautiful world".

"There is great who never fails but one who never gives up. Thank you for giving us so much! ".

Cristo Delgado,
Coach Personal, Nutrition Advisory
Spain

"My trips are always full of moments that I remember with the heart and with love, Valentín has done something very big, sharing and helping us to learn more about health and personal well-being".

Gabriela Rivero,
Degree in Education
Travel & Tourism Professional model, @ecoviajeravzla
Venezuela

"I could highlight many facets and qualities of Valentín López is very clear that loves to inform and motivate. This time with this book, very comprehensive and structured that serves as a practical guide to learn how to improve our physical and mental health, both user and professional ".

Naira Bolaños,
Personal Trainer, Competitor IFBB Wellness
Spain

"You read *How to take care of yourself for success* and it's like you finish first in a marathon. Dreams are to achieve them but you have to work with them and with Valentín López you have a great support and push. Thank you!".

Kiko Barroso,
Radiophonic Journalist
Presenter of *Roscas and Cotufas* in the Canary Islands Radio Co-presenter the *Canarias Today* on TV Canaria
Spain

"What I most appreciate this amazing adventure is to meet wonderful people. One of the things that motivated me to read *How to take care of yourself for success* is the personality of Valentín, I firmly believe that when you know where you're going, until the world turns aside to let you pass, this is the case of Valentín always helping and granting it better humanity. I thank God for giving me the opportunity to meet you, I highly recommend reading as it has been of great benefit to me".

"I've loved, I know you will continue to achieve many successes to share with others".

Efrén García,
Communicator and dreams Producer Digital Marketing,
@coachviajero
Venezuela

"If we do not discipline ourselves to be healthy in body and mind nothing will prepare in other areas. This is the phrase that came to mind after reading *How to take care of yourself for success*. Valentín López has not only been a constant source of inspiration and motivation on the path to success but now gives us the possibility of be physically and mentally prepared to enjoy. As Chef this book made me remember that food has a more important and deeper than meet an immediate need objective. I have been fascinated and now form part of my personal computer to consult when preparing menus ".

Andrew Reyes,
Chef International Cuisine
Dominican Republic

"In the West, I have much to discover and learn about medicinal plants and nutritional principles, Valentín has managed to harmonize in this book, the balance between the mind and the basic influences of life, such as body and food".

"You will always be welcome to my temple friend".

Ryoshun Seike,
Buddhist Monk
Traditional Medicine, Ayurveda, *ryoshun.com*
India

"I loved reading How to care for success, without a doubt Valentín is a blessing for our country, congratulations for this great book, I am very excited. Much success my friend! ".

Madalena Rodrigues,
Entrepreneur
Brazil

"I met Valentín when I invited him to one of my projects, the program *The Friday Armchair*, I was surprised by his positivity in the face of adversity and much more, his advice on the attitude we have to take in any circumstance. As Valentín says; Success resides in us! Congratulations for this great project".

Florentín Díaz,
Journalist, Event Presenter
Television Image
Spain

"To get the things you never thought to have, you need to do things you never thought you could do. When you put passion and dedication it shows, *How to take care of yourself for success* is a great example. I'm very proud of you Valentín".

"You are not what you achieve, you are what you surpass".

Sabina Herrera,
Teacher, Sports Nutritionist
Trainer Bikini, Mens Physique, Wellness
Spain

"It's amazing the things we can learn with this great book by Valentín, *How to take care of yourself for success* will teach you many of them that you can not miss".

Lidiane Alves,
Psychologist, Business Woman
Restorante O Caipira
Brazil

"I am sure that this book will help many to get to know each other better. Grateful with your friendship always Valentín".

Fabian Fitzner,
Speaker, Public Image, Businessman
Dubai, United Arab Emirates

"Valentín López is a great friend, an example of overcoming, perseverance, growth and, above all, the desire to add value to others, which is why I always say that people like him have to be close to them. Taking care of yourself for success fills you with awareness, habits and, above all, pillars of our nature to provide health and well-being".

"Congratulations for the value and benefit you give to society in this book, I loved it".

Miguel Reus,
Businessman
Spain

"How to take care of yourself for success is just another example of how Valentín López continues to empower people around the world". "Thanks for sharing this with me Valentín".

Daniela Miron,
Businesswoman
Romania

"I love health, this book gives you clear instructions on how to help you in your next goals". "I loved reading it, friend Valentín great project".

Mary Grace Zaragoza
Businesswoman, Sales Agent
Financial Consultant
Philippines

"Today, success is more within reach than ever, I am the living example coming from a country that they call without resources and now I manage six-figure businesses. It takes focus, intelligence and hardness, but not before achieving good health and physical care. How to take care of yourself for success reveals exact, simple, simple and super effective steps. These are the small details that will give you a competitive advantage to achieve the dreams you want".

"Everything is possible if you really believe in yourself".

Josue Pena,
CEO Founder Digital
Dominican Republic

"You have opened my mind Valentín simple and very well classified, this book gives us practical solutions to know where to start to improve. Whoever follows the instructions of *How to take care of yourself for success* in the way you are here explained will radically change your life".

Joseph Lai,
Entrepreneur
Malaysia

"Since I read *How to take care of yourself for success*, I knew that I was going to make it very easy for the world to improve their lifestyle. Valentín knows how to adapt the complex and turn it into useful information. Great communicator of his message and an entire influence".

Joe Stewart,
Author of Self Publishing Empire
Editor in Chief of TheWashingtonInsider.com
USA

WORDS OF JACOBO CASTILLO

"Those who call us crazy are those who do not have the courage to fight for their dreams, but do you know what Valentine? where some see a madman, others see a talented young man, armed with wisdom for battle, temperance in the dark and a source of inexhaustible inspiration to be able to mobilize any army. Your energized words can raise any deity, that's your skill, my friend".

"Another crazy man in a world of saps, here lost in Macaronesia. You have a General prepared to accompany you, together we are stronger".

"Do not forget this Valentín; who has magic does not need tricks".

Jacobo Castillo,
CEO Canary Group
Visionary
Spain

INTRODUCTION

This book is about one of the areas most important to me: the personal well-being and physical care. I consider it an issue as sufficiently valuable to take the time to write about it.

Here you will find a brief narrative, very practical and simple guide on supplements, plants and nutritional principles embodied experience, self-improvement, constant learning and working hard and smart with fiery intended to help you classify, group and be better informed about your choice in the different market advantages and nature can offer you depending on their sport needs or health reasons.

Warning: Proceed with consistency, monitoring your personal needs by weight, somatotype and diagnostics about your health. Please before making a decision, lean on your doctor, nutritionist, fi physiotherapist or personal sports coach for an individual assessment and which will create the best diet plan and training to measure, by modifying the guidelines that they deem necessary.

And remember this: to trust in oneself is the key to achieving resilience and overcome adversity pillar, stop to ask if you have talent or not, Strive to improve every day in your area and I'll see you getting it!

See you in the winner's circle.

Valentín López

The opposite of success is not failure as many people think, are the excuses and conformism submerged in a vacuum of purpose that feed it. Please do not pass that, you're not to meet just one time, you're to fulfill your dreams!

FIRST PART

1. INCREASE IN PROTEIN SYNTHESIS AND MUSCLE ANABOLISM

Whey Protein: One of the basic supplements that you can use in your physical activity is the whey or fermented milk products. It is composed of essential and nonessential amino acids. Select it as filter system (concentrated, isolated, hydrolyzed, mixtures, etc.) since its value depends on the amount of sugars and amino acids (particularly the amount of Leucine) to house as the seriousness of their diet. Some are already enriched with more BCAAs, glutamine, creatine and even vitamins to improve absorption. Nah moment of decision? None, but because of its rapid absorption may be of interest immediately after waking up, about physical activity or before bedtime. Everything will depend on the daily and weekly intake of protein supplement and not a sole factor.

And according to studies generally from 0.9 grams per kilo of weight in adulthood and can enjoy its benefits. Several authors and recent research agree intake for athletes based on an average of 1.2-2 grams per kilo of weight. Also in the market you can find supplements of meat protein for intolerant or those who suffer different conditions. Add or delete the number of outlets to reach your daily protein requirements. Remember greater nitrogen retention in the short term may reflect a greater increase in protein however for an individual to take more excess protein does not imply increased protein synthesis. Many of the protein products today are overrated, do not neglect your eating plan with the excuse to include more supplements. shots are recommended 20-30 grams food however has shown that people who put up 70% of protein in one meal do not lose muscle mass. Careful when ingesting hot liquids supplement whey protein with these mixed as "could" denature affecting their biological properties. Always act with congruence adapting your eating plan the number of meals daily grams of macronutrients and calories. Lean on his nutritionist.

What you will find below is a list of essential amino acids that will benefit in his health. "Essential" means that in order to exploit their properties and benefits, must be ingested through food (such as meat, fish, legumes, cereals, dairy products, eggs ...) or supplements.

ESSENTIAL AMINO ACIDS

BCAAs: They appear here because they are composed of a trio of essential amino acids. They are rami fi ed because they provide energy when oxidized in the body. These are: leucine, isoleucine, valine. normally used to reduce fatigue and wear in training. It is recommended to take before and after physical activity (3-20 grams / day) with whey protein to increase the synthesis. If several doses per day is required are taking them at least 15-10 minutes before meals as they could compete with other amino acids in absorption. They are easily digested. It may be better assimilation through intake of vitamin B6, vitamin C, zinc, chromium and magnesium.

Leucine: Together with the L-isoleucine and growth hormone (HGH), interferes with the formation and repair of muscle tissue. For people who make a large number of meals per day may bene fi ciarles an extra supply of leucine to maximize the amount of protein ingested. (CDR: 14 mg / kg).

Isoleucine: Beyond intervening processes muscle tissue repair provides benefits for oxygenating the circulatory system improving CO2 transport blood through hemoglobin (quaternary protein that allows the transport of oxygen) regulating the levels of blood glucose. (CDR: 10 mg / kg).

Valine: It stimulates growth, repair and tissue healing, maintenance of various systems and is involved in nitrogen balance. (CDR: 10 mg / kg).

Lysine: It is one of the most important amino acids because, in association with several amino acids more involved in various functions, including growth, tissue repair, and immune system antibodies hormone synthesis. Studies suggest that lysine ingested L-carnitine, helps lower blood cholesterol levels. Lysine turn stimulates the release of growth hormone. Interesting combination with arginine. (Lysine intake is around 12 milligrams per kilo of body weight).

Methionine: Powerful antioxidant and a good source of sulfur for the body. It is an intermediate in the biosynthesis of cysteine, carnitine, taurine, lecithin, phosphatidylcholine and other phospholipids. Failures in the conversion of methionine can lead to atherosclerosis. It is responsible for transporting fat into the cells for energy, and achieve better muscle performance. In this passage of body fat which makes this amino acid is to prevent the accumulation of it in the arteries and liver, and thus achieve good physical health at various levels. Sulfur content contribute helps improve joint cartilage. (CDR: 13 mg / kg).

Tryptophan: It is involved in the growth and hormone production, especially in the function of the glands of adrenal secretion. Responsible for the production of serotonin (a neurotransmitter that controls our mood, relaxation and sleep). It helps the formation of GABA (gamma aminobutyric acid) neurotransmitter widely distributed in neurons of the cerebral cortex. Promotes the release of growth hormone. (CDR: 3.5 mg / Kg).

Phenylalanine: Involved in the production of collagen, mainly in the structure of the skin and connective tissue, and also in the formation of several neurohormones. As endogenous has analgesic properties to reduce muscle pain. Synthesizes the amino acid tyrosine. Present in the process of producing melanin for hair and skin. Releases endorphins. Alleviate the pain. Beware because its excess is included with aspartic acid and many sweetener in many soft drinks and medicines for its power to sweeten and flavor. See contraindications with your doctor. (CDR: 14 mg / kg).

Threonine: Along with the L-methionine and aspartic acid, helps the liver in its general detoxification functions (fatty liver disorder). It facilitates the absorption of nutrients. Participates in the formation of collagen, elastin and enamel teeth. It helps protect against intestinal infections. Aids digestion. Improves liver function. (CDR: 7 mg / kg).

After studying and classifying essential and discover amino acids that must be provided externally and which are vital for our body we present the list of "non-essential" amino acids, and that the body can synthesize by itself or from other amino acids without the need for direct intake.

NON ESSENTIAL AMINO ACIDS

Alanine amino acid: Involved in the metabolism of glucose, tryptophan and Vitamin B6. It helps stabilize blood sugar levels. In addition to its benefits as a source of natural energy, it helps metabolize both organic acids such as sugar.

Arginine: It is involved in the maintenance of equilibrium nitrogen and carbon dioxide. It also has a great importance in the production of growth hormone directly involved in the growth of tissues and muscles and in the maintenance and repair of the immune system. It reduces body fat levels and facilitates recovery of athletes due to the effects of removing ammonia (resulting residue anaerobic exercise muscle) of muscles and convert urea that is excreted in urine. It is often used before physical activity or before bedtime. Interesting combination with lysine. Check with your doctor.

Asparagine: Specific intervenes in the metabolic processes of the central nervous system (CNS). Precursor of GABA.

Aspartic acid: Involved in protein processing within the Krebs cycle. It is very important for liver detoxification and proper operation. This amino combined with other amino acid molecules forming capases

absorb toxins from the bloodstream. It has proven to be a stimulator in the release of luteinizing hormone (LH) and growth hormone (GH) from the pituitary gland. (Luteinizing hormone LH, is the chemical messenger that travels from the pituitary to the testicles, where testosterone production is activated).
Participates in the formation of glutamic acid or glutamate. Widely used as a supplement for increased muscle tone, expelling ammonia, cleanse the blood and prevent fatigue.

Citrulline: Despite being a non-protein amino, it is an intermediate in the synthesis of the amino acid arginine. Participates in the urea cycle, which intervenes mechanism by speci fi c in removing ammonia and toxic substances from the body through urine. It produces beneficial effects on the heart, circulatory system and bene fi ts the immune system. It is widely marketed as citrulline malate to enhance athletic performance, as has been shown in preliminary clinical trials, which reduces muscle fatigue. Recommended physical activity before or at bedtime to recover. It can also be found abundantly in watermelon, where it was first isolated.

Cysteine: It is manufactured from methionine. L-cysteine is involved in detoxification, mainly as free radical antagonist. Because cysteine can be easily oxidized cystine is preferred stable form of L-cysteine, N-acetylcysteine (NAC), for nutritional supplements. NAC also form glutathione, which is a combination of three amino acids: cysteine, glycine and glutamic acid, (called "tripeptide"). Glutathione is one of the most powerful antioxidants and protects cells against oxidative stress. It also helps maintain healthy hair because of its high sulfur content and its antioxidant action. It helps eliminate heavy metals. It helps detoxify the bowel. It acts as a potent mucolytic aiding the elimination of dense mucus airway. Prevent cataracts, retinal decay. Detoxifies the liver cells and the lymphatic system. Relieves arthritis. It stabilizes blood sugar. Protects the digestive system. Consult your doctor.

Cystine: It is created by two cysteines. Also it involved in detoxification, in combination with the above amino acid. The L-cystine is very important in the synthesis of insulin and in the reactions of certain molecules to this.

Glutamine: It represents almost 60% of total amino acids in the muscles. It has ergogenic effect of repair of muscle fibers. Crosses the blood-brain barrier becoming glutamic acid, thereby raising the concentration thereof in the brain. Its use supports neutralize excess lactic acid (Buffer effect) in the muscles. Prevents loss of muscle mass. With alanine transport more than half of the nitrogen in the body. Helps cleanse the ammonia from the body so his recommendation after physical activity or at night. It could help prevent muscle loss during long idle times. It contributes to the formation of GABA (gamma-aminobutyric acid). The results could be bene fi cial especially when there is deficiency of this amino acid. Consult your specialist.

Glutamic Acid (Glutamate): It has great importance in the functioning of the central nervous system and acts as an immune system stimulant. Carries amino acids and nitrogen. It helps in the production of hydrochloric acid (to improve digestion). Controlling ammonia levels in the brain. Excellent in the treatment of normal prostate function. Precursor of GABA. It plays a fundamental role in maintaining and cell growth. Precursor for the synthesis of nucleic acids (DNA). Prevents intestinal atrophy and infections. Reduces intestinal permeability. Regulates the production of urea in the liver. It leads to an increase in growth hormone, which helps maintain muscle mass. Consult your doctor and your deficit may hold in memory problems, learning and loss of reflexes.

Glycine: You require the presence of serine (another amino acid) for their manufacture. It increases the absorption of creatine. It helps control ammonia levels in the brain. tranquilizing neurotransmitter in the brain. It helps increase the release of growth hormone. Retards muscle degeneration. Heals wounds, fractures, dislocations and damaged tissues. It promotes a healthy prostate. It helps store glycogen. Retards muscle breakdown. Involved in the production of collagen and phospholipids.

Histidine: Essential in children and in adults not essential. In combination with growth hormone (HGH), contribute to the development to adulthood. Cardio-protective and vasodilator. It helps heal wounds. Treats rheumatoid arthritis and improves digestion. It plays a key role in neuronal functioning, causing the strengthening of synapses (electrical impulses) in the brain where it is needed. Precursor histamine regulates the immune response to pathogens, harmful bacteria and viruses. Histidine deficiency is characterized by hearing loss and difficulty to repair tissues. It is often used as a complement to increase tissue regeneration of the skin and accelerate the recovery of muscle injuries. Increased levels of carnosine with this amino acid provides greater control over the acidosis produced by exercise.

Serine: From serine you can perform the synthesis of other amino acids such as tryptophan, glycine and cysteine. metabolism of fats and fatty acids. Controls cholesterol absorption. It helps the production of immunoglobulins and antibodies. Necessary for muscle growth, the formation of cells and antibodies. It can contribute to improving physical performance and muscle recovery after exercise taken.

Taurine: Recognized mainly because part of certain energy drinks popularidad.Estimula growth hormone (HGH). Involved in the regulation of blood pressure, strengthens the heart muscle and energizes the nervous system. Delay fatigue. Improves vision and helps prevent macular degeneration. It is the key component of bile, which is necessary for fat digestion, useful for people with arteriosclerosis, edema, heart disorders, hypertension or hypoglycemia. Prevents heart problems, increases the power of the heart, blood pressure decreases. Antidepressant. Regulates diabetes. It facilitates physical recovery. It facilitates the transport of oxygen and creatine. Reduces the production of ammonia during physical exertion. GABA increases the effects of lowering anxiety and stress. Carnosine and taurine increases muscle strength to counteract the muscle cell action causing byproducts of fatigue. You can contribute meal plans and weight loss workouts because of its activation.

Tyrosine: Synthesized from phenylalanine. Antidepressant and anti stress. It is a precursor of epinephrine and dopamine, (a substance closely related mood states) and melanin (skin pigment). It is usually complemented tyrosine because it suppresses appetite and helps reduce body fat. Next to iodine is required for the manufacture of thyroid hormones. It stimulates the release of growth hormone which may lead to increased muscle mass depending on protein synthesis. Potentiates the activity and mental concentration.

Ornithine: Precursor of arginine. Growth hormone releasing (HGH). Helps the metabolism of body fat (this effect is greater when combined with arginine and L-carnitine). It promotes healing by stimulating collagen synthesis. Intoxications, bene fi cal function and liver regeneration. Fl ows in the synthesis of insulin in the pancreas. It promotes the removal of ammonia through the liver, through the urea cycle. If arginine is taken is usually taken in a ratio of 2: 1 being for example 2 grams per 1 gram of arginine ornithine. (Before bedtime or during physical activity).

Proline: It is essential for the restoration and healing of damaged connective tissues. Helps in the treatment of joint diseases. It contributes to improving skin texture, helping collagen production and reduce its loss through the aging process. As part of the cartilage aid in healing and strengthening the joints, tendons and heart muscles. Proline works with vitamin C to help maintain healthy connective tissues. It acts as a cardiovascular protective, inhibiting the decomposition of collagen blood, to thereby prevent possible injury. It can contribute its improvement in certain injuries (meniscus cartilage connections ...) when combined with supplements such as glucosamine, chondroitin or MSM "methylsulfonylmethane".

What we have seen so far it is a classification of essential and nonessential amino acids showing the benefits of each and major improvements to your health. What then will read several add-ons that suggest interesting for physical activity, and intends to improve muscle mass, reduce catabolism (protein breakdown) or speed recovery or support any of efficiency.

HMB (Beta-hydroxy beta-methylbutyrate): Acid that exists naturally in the body (produce an average of 0.2 to 0.4 grams of HMB per day depending on the ingested leucine) when the amino acid leucine decomposes, (integral BCAA), therefore, that it has been shown to stimulate protein synthesis through mTOR / p70S6k. Reduces cortisol and body fat. Prevents enzymes break muscle tissue for energy production. Avoids catabolism by disrupting proteolysis (natural process of decomposition of muscle tissue which occurs after intense physical activity). HMB supplementation has been very effective in lowering LDL cholesterol (*Nissen, 2000*). Increases maximum oxygen consumption (VO2 max) and improves respiratory compensation point (RCP). Recent studies suggest that HMB may reduce metabolic acidosis, blood lactate and ammonia, which could improve recovery but need clarification of an effort much deeper investigation.

Phosphatidylserine: Formed by two molecules of fatty acid and nonessential amino acid serine. Phospholipid determines the integrity and the fluidity of cell membranes (particularly the brain) there being attributed a special ability to improve memory (because it synthesizes acetylcholine, a type of neurotransmitter with high relevance in memory short term), the translation of the signals (cause the correct functioning of brain organs such as the cortex, hypothalamus and pituitary gland), release of the secretory vesicles and regulation cell growth. It is often used after training by reducing cortisol and muscle pain in addition to speed recovery. A study shows that 800 mg of phosphatidylserine taken in divided oral doses, suppresses cortisol caused by intense weight training. It is usually combined with the

Omega-3 400-500 mg phosphatidylserine although the standard dose is 300 mg divided 3 times. Consult your doctor and your deficit is related to Alzheimer's, Parkinson's, multiple sclerosis and ADHD.

One of the main causes of increased cortisol is anxiety, nervous stomach and chest pressure generated stress. Testosterone levels tend to decline causing fatigue and nervousness, so it might be interesting to take supplements of phosphatidylserine at night. Numerous cases have been reported markedly reduced anxiety the next day. You can also find it in soy, egg yolk, livers and beans but it may be insufficient. Find good about it.

Coenzyme Q10 (ubiquinone): It is a well known potent antioxidant that helps protect against damage from free radicals, and is involved in cellular energy production. Therefore it is essential for the functioning of almost every cell .. participates in aerobic cellular respiration, generating energy in the form of ATP. Ninety-five percent of the human body's energy is generated this way. Therefore, the organs with higher energy requirement (such as the heart and liver) are those with higher concentrations of coenzyme Q10. It can be found in mackerel, herring, tuna, sardines, salmon, soybeans, peanuts, eggs, seeds, livers and hearts of pork and beef. In one study I read *The Journal of Urology* 2012 the positive effects of ubiquinol in patients with male infertility were published. Usually comes added especially multivitamins and supplements for sport because it increases oxygen utilization by our body, has anti-aging properties and increases the immune system's ability to fight disease. Doses averaged 10-20 mg. Read more about it and consult with professionals.

Beta-Alanine (3-aminopropanoic acid): Non essential amino acid that is usually combined with creatine before training. While beta-alanine increases the pH and therefore reduces muscle fatigue, creatine aid in ATP synthesis, so also increases energy levels. Basically beta-alanine increases carnosine levels inhibits this effect causes excess lactic acid delaying fatigue. So it's ideal for strength athletes or muscle deve-lopment. It can be found in meat and fish. Doses vary from 0.02 g / kg to 0.05 g / kg daily. Carefully document about it.

Betaine (trimethylglycine),: It has been included in many pre-workout supplements for their benefits on athletic performance. Choline is a precursor of betaine, the synthesized with the amino acid glycine. Where first isolated it was in beet (hence its Latin name). In a good "pre-training" home it is usually mixed with caffeine, creatine, beta-alanine, citrulline malate and arginine as betaine increases vascularity and vasodilator effect, improving circulation in the bloodstream (and supporting the absorption of BCAAs in the case of also be ingested). Apart from increasing the strength and endurance and reduce muscle fatigue. Doses vary depending on body composition and the training of 500 to 2500 milligrams.

Creatine: Probably no other supplement has been more studied than creatine. It is a nitrogenous organic acid found in muscle and nerve cells. It is synthesized in the liver, pancreas, kidneys from three amino acids: arginine, glycine and methionine. Creatine is one of the most used in the sport as it is a direct and immediate to regenerate ATP and provide energy supplements muscle cells source. greater volume, to favor the increase of muscle glycogen and water retention intracellular optimizing protein synthesis is achieved.

Improves glucose control, prevent bone loss and muscle weakness and improve cognitive ability. The recommendations point to 0.08 gr./kilo. Generally distributed before and / or after training. There are studies that show that the combining creatine with a simple carbohydrate increases transport this into the muscle. Vegetarians can bene fi t even oral administration of creatine. Keep in mind that one gram of muscle glycogen stored is attached to about 3 grams of water so if during a charging phase of the body carbohydrate stores 300-400 grams additional glycogen, together with those of 900-1200 grams water increase body weight about 1200-1600 grams above normal. This must be taken into account especially in weight loss diets with carbohydrate restriction as the first kilos you lose water retention is due to decreased glycogen. Carefully document about it and consult your specialist.

Beef liver tablets: This supplement has been for a long time in sport and not only in intense preparations but also in aerobics. Liver tablets provide organic iron, protein and vitamin B complex plus amino acids, vitamins and minerals. Iron is vital for growth in sport because it is necessary to manufacture two major proteins in the body: hemoglobin, a constituent of blood cells that provides the red color and myoglobin, a protein that carries oxygen muscle cells. Read carefully if you have iron deficiencies because they can be altered globules blood instead of increasing their share, if nutrition is not correct.

Carbohydrates different absorption and digestion: There are many supplements on the market such as dextrose, vitargo, GLUT-4 among others because they are absorbed immediately by the body, providing muscles extra energy that helps a more intense physical exercise and replenish glycogen stores. Also Carefully document polysaccharides slower absorption such as the amylopectin or maltodextrins exercise longer lasting as cross fi t, running, tennis, football ... It is usually given when glucose levels are low, plans feed volume its extracalórico and mobilizing other supplements input, such as whey protein or creatine. (Since the insulin peak increase more substances are mobilized within the cell).

The shots often vary but a fairly accurate indicator usually between 0.2-0.8 kilo grams obviously depending on the objectives and seeks to achieve caloric settings of your eating plan. It can even be used for different types of recovery honey, propolis and royal jelly (in addition to those being loaded with antioxidants, vitamins and minerals). Many football players usually take before bedtime two tablespoons of apple vinegar and honey dissolved in a cup of hot water scoops. Many athletes noticed an increase in strength and recovery.

If you have some toxic people around you are bothered
by chance and let them
know, sorry, your success
will pay them the psycho-
logist but remember: your
happiness is not negotiable.

2. STIMULATION IN THE OXIDATION OF FATS WITH THE SUPPORT OF THE CALORIC DEFICIT

I'll tell you something you probably already know, besides good physical activity, have low levels of fat and have a flatter belly and fi nest are made in the kitchen. That is, a good diet plan to control the calories and with macro- and micronutrients ruled by your specialist will be vital to its success. Even so, and with this in mind and in mind, we present below a series of additions that could bene fi ciarle in that extra loss (directly or indirectly) fat while composing your meals and workout plan.

L-Carnitine Used primarily for performance, recovery and reducing fat loss when accompanied with caloric fi cit as it deals with transport fatty acids into the mitochondria.

There are several studies in the sport in which you can increase the benefits (especially when supplemented with fatty acids like fish) and when there is deficit. Ask your doctor maintain good levels of insulin as in definitive, lipid layer of a cell is basically composed of omega 3 fatty acids, the cell will also be more sensitive to this, which will allow his body more energy.

L-carnitine is synthesized in the liver, kidneys and brain from two essential amino acids, lysine and methionine. "Amine" (organic chemical compound which is considered as derived from ammonia) that helps better mitochondria oxidize fatty acids and produce ATP (adenosine triphosphate). Acetyl L-carnitine occurs abundantly in the brain and prevent cell aging. It can also be combined with tyrosine plans weight loss because it suppresses appetite and helps reduce body fat when caloric fi cit is followed. And with serine (since this amino acid affects the metabolism of fats and fatty acids) and L-methionine (responsible for transporting fat to the cells to oxidize energy. Furthermore, the function of L-methionine is helping to prevent the accumulation of fat in the arteries and liver. Study the benefits of L-carnitine because it can improve athletic performance, speed recovery after intense exercise, reduce accumulation of lactic acid in muscle and contribute to improve brain function and help prevent oxidative stress that can lead to long term health problems such as cardiovascular disease, diabetes and chronic inflammation. It can be supplemented with other nutrients such as zinc, vitamin C, B6, B12 and the amino acid L-arginine. See also your cardiologist. If female consult your obstetrician if you are pregnant because there are also studies in which the contribution of L-carnitine may be a small help in cardiovascular functions and benefits for the heart during exercise and recovery, since it intervenes in the blood pressure, oxygen supply and muscle contraction bene fi ciándose each other. The therapeutic dose ranges from 500-2000 mg daily. Put yourself in the hands of your doctor and nutritionist before making a decision.

MCT: The main reason to use MCT supplement is being used by ketones (derived from stored or ingested fats) as an energy source and is not deposited as fat in the body. According to its acronym, medium chain triglycerides comprise 6-12 carbons and are naturally in coconut oil, as well as dairy products like milk, butter and cheese. Most sources of fat consumed are made of long-chain triglycerides (LCT), digested differently from the MCT as these are manufactured by isolating these medium-chain triglycerides of other triglycerides and then packaged being used as a complement.

The body processes differently MCT LCT, The shorter the carbon chain, more efficient will be the MCT ketones, (these produce less reactive oxygen because they are metabolized to produce ATP). He coconut oil It has a mixture of all medium-chain fats (between 60% - 70% of its weight is MCT), including fats C6, C8, C10 and C12, however, caprylic fatty acid (C8) and capric (C10) MCT levels rise more and ketones sufficiently since become mitochondrial fuel. Ketones also help suppress ghrelin (hormone hunger synthesized by the stomach). The MCT acts differently from long chain fatty feeding in (LCT) manner, fat taken from the body must be mixed with bile released from the gallbladder, and pancreatic enzymes to be decomposed by the digestive system. But MCT is different because it does not need bile nor pancreatic enzymes need. (So it is interesting in people with stomach or malabsorption of fat) problems. Once the MCT into the intestine, are directed through the intestinal membrane into the blood stream and are moved directly to the liver, where the oil becomes ketones. Liver subsequently released ketones back into the bloodstream where it is transported throughout the body. (Even can pass the blood brain barrier to provide power to the brain). It has a thermogenic effect, creating an effect positive for metabolism. So they are easily utilized by the body, because they generate energy (fuel instead of carbohydrates), rather than being stored as fat. Check with your doctor. Take the MCT slowly to tolerate feedings. Studies suggest an ideal concentration of ketones for maximum suppression of hunger and fat burning 0.48 millimoles per liter (mmol / L). (Beta hydroxybutyrate levels as blood glucose are measured). If you want to deepen, ketones measurements can be performed through urine, breath or blood tests. I have found that many athletes to lose fat usually they enter ketosis doing two to three days of fasting a month taking on rising oil MCT (three times a day and doses every 4 hours) with caprylic acid (C8). Exogenous ketones help meet the anguish of momentary lack of carbohydrates. Once you enter ketosis the body will use its endogenous much fat. To maintain this state the aim is to consume enough fat (1 to 1.5 grams per kilo of body weight) and 1 to 1.5 grams of protein. Too little fat and protein has not worked since the liver converts the excess amino acids into glucose, ending ketosis. In the process usually mixed with coconut milk coffee in a thermos to take between meals and keep high doses of fat. Use with caution these temporary methods and rely on his trainer or nutritionist.

Chitosan: In short this add is that it could be a "natural fat sensor". It comes from chitin found in the skeletons of crustaceans. It has the ability to bind fats and cholesterol in the digestive tract before they can be absorbed by the body. Therefore it is used in thousands of food preparations and dozens of marketing products for thinning. A good way to ingest it is before meals. It is interesting because it can help control cholesterol levels (LDL) and blood pressure. Often combined with other products such as glucomannan, carob or Garcinia cambogia (also explained in this book) for use in controlling appetite and weight loss.

Inositol and Choline: You can find them especially in energy drinks and commercial slimming supplements. Despite being considered members of the B vitamins we decided to include them in this section. Inositol has the ability to mobilize fatty acids as energy to oxidize also preventing its accumulation in liver tissues. Choline is needed for transporting cholesterol from the liver. The deficiency of choline may cause excessive accumulation of fat and cholesterol. Also it helps omega-3 fatty acids and vitamins B and D (so can be complemented). If female study hill at times of pregnancy and lactation because it is important to maintain good levels (as folic acid).

Hill also has uses for studies on the brain (Alzheimer ...) and heart Carefully document so professional about it. You can find it in a variety of meats and vegetables, fish, egg yolks ... (only two whole eggs a day provide half the hill "most" people need). Inositol can get in lecithin, wheat germ, oatmeal, beef liver, nuts and legumes. Also consider direct effects on hair, skin, nails, reducing cholesterol, symptoms of anxiety and stress and cardiovascular activity.

Do not let fear paralyze you, demotivate you and make you back. Even afraid you have to act, that indicates bravery, courage and determination, and not by the absence of this precisely. Just prepare yourself and become bigger! for fear you no longer matters.

3. THE VALUE OF VITAMINS AND MINERALS

Although a varied diet is usually rich in itself in vitamins and minerals, depending on physical activity chosen and the approach of eating plan can sometimes be some deficiency states which can trigger many diseases in the body, fatigue and tiredness. The good news is you can get them from specific food or as supplements. Depending on your country and your personal issues always check the new editions of the RDA (Recommended Daily Allowance) and CDDSAE (Dietary Allowance and Adequate Insurance Dear Diary) established by the *National Academy of Sciences,* he *National Research* or the *Food and Nutrition Board.* Some organizations such as the World Health Organization (WHO) and the Food and Agriculture Organization (FAO) recomputed and determine the amount each nutrient should be consumed in the diet plan. However the RDA is not appropriate for some individuals who have very specific nutritional needs (especially in amino acids, vitamins or minerals) due to sport or their health diagnoses. Remember that there will be some marketing behind multivitamins, it is best to be selective after a blood test because many contain large amounts of what you do not need and very few of those who did. Keeping this in mind. Here's a brief guide to express these organic compounds to give you an idea of their benefits and contribution. Since they are considered essential in food with carbohydrates, proteins, fats and water.

Vitamin A (Retinol): After the liver, the tissue more stores this vitamin is the retina of the eye. The safest way to take it is in the form of beta-carotene because it is a precursor of vitamin A. Increase immunity protects radiation and is preventive in chronic diseases, and infectious organism helping the healing of tissues.

This powerful antioxidant and anticarcinogenic (only carotenes and Xantorows) also has benefits to the skin maintaining hydration and elasticity. Improves the condition of the cartilage, bone and teeth as well as being an indispensable part of the vision (pigments in the retina of the eye). You can find it in much greater quantity in the livers and its derivatives, carrots, turnips, spinach, sweet potatoes, cabbage, pumpkin, lettuce, chard, red pepper, tomatoes, butter, hard cheese, egg yolks and tuna.

B vitamins: Also commonly they found in supplement form together all of them. Most do not produce them so they must be ingested for the proper functioning of the body:

Vitamin B1 (Thiamine): It is essential for the functioning of the nervous system and also acts as a coenzyme in energy production from carbohydrates.

Vitamin B2 (Ribo fl avina): Energy production, antioxidant, and nervous system tissue regeneration. Part of the retina and potency vitamin E.

Vitamin B3 (Niacin): Metabolism of carbohydrates, proteins and fats into energy. nervous, muscular, circulatory and cardiac system. Control of sleep. It may occur through the amino acid tryptophan. Necessary for healthy skin.

Vitamin B5 (Pantothenic Acid): Metabolizes macronutrient energy involved in adrenaline and insulin, formation of erythrocytes and oxygen transport.

Vitamin B6 (pyridoxine) Coenzyme in the metabolism of proteins, creating hemoglobin in the blood, nervous and immune system. Very important in the absorption of amino acids and glycogenolysis (breakdown of glycogen to glucose) and gluconeogenesis (glucose biosynthesis from precursors glucidic not).

Vitamin B7, B8 (Biotin): Vitamin B5 power. Macronutrient metabolism. Involved in the system nervous, blood hemoglobin and glycolysis (oxidation of glucose for energy). Say that pyruvate is the product resulting from glycolysis: in sport conditions oxygen is transformed into acetyl-CoA while anaerobically becomes lactic acid.

Vitamin B9 (folic acid or): Involved in the production of DNA (genetic material) and RNA (protein formation and cell processes). Also interesting if women during periods of pregnancy because their requirements are higher.

Vitamin B12 (cyanocobalamin): It is not found in any plant product without embrago not all of animal origin are rich in B12. Involved in the functioning of the brain, nervous system and metabolism of proteins, fats and carbohydrates as well as DNA synthesis. Interesting is its extra contribution especially when it is a strict vegetarian since these may suffer from deficiencies of this vitamin.

Have to know that usually sell complex with several vitamins together the group B to which is added choline and inositol (those involved in the formation of cell membranes, lipid metabolism and brain neurotransmitters, cholesterol regulation and system digestive). Also, if you are a woman, you should know that vitamin B9 along with choline are very important for the formation of the fetus during pregnancy. Get advice from professional.

Vitamin C (ascorbic acid): It is a powerful antioxidant with great importance for normal growth and development of our organism. Promotes absorption of iron, formation of collagen and adrenaline.

Vitamin D (calciferol), D2 (ergocalciferol and D3 (calciferol): Vitamin D increases the absorption of calcium and phosphorus in the small intestine fi fixing it in bones and teeth. You can be obtained from foods, supplements or transformation cholesterol or ergosterol due to exposure to sunlight (production D2 and D3).

Vitamin E (Tocopherol): Antirust. Involved in the circulatory system and heart cholesterol regulation. Promotes creatine transport to the muscles for subsequent production of energy (ATP).

Vitamin K: Processes involved in blood clotting, regulating cholesterol and indirectly in the calcification in the bones.

Remember that the water soluble vitamins such as the B and C complex are easily excreted through urine when there is excess. (The body does not have a reservation meaningful of these vitamins, except of C) while the fat-soluble (A, D, E, and K) are dissolved in fat (absorbed lipoprotein) can be stored in the fatty tissue of organism so be careful with the latter because their excess through aggressive supplementation may have different ailments over the weeks.

If we stop to read the advertising of vitamin supplements do us the idea that it is very difficult to obtain an adequate supply of vitamins from food plan. Conversely entities such as the *American Medical Association* or the *National Research Council* believe that a plan over 1500 calories and is balanced is more than enough to meet the needs of the individual. However there is some truth in both positions because the power of certain people if they may be unbalanced and then bene fi t from these supplements could be paramount.

MACROMINERALS

Minerals are an essential source for the body and I will be guided by some of these inorganic elements and which in turn are the most important ones are usually supplemented if deficiencies or higher requirements for physical activity as we cited above.

Magnesium: Fi jar helps calcium and phosphorus in bones and teeth. It could prevent kidney stones because it mobilizes calcium. It also acts as a mild laxative and antacid. Tranquilizer and natural antidepressant. It helps produce and release GABA one of the major inhibitory neurotransmitters for sleep. His deficiency may be associated with muscle cramps.

Calcium: Hydration with vitamin D is very important to increase the absorption of this mineral. The most important function of calcium is building bones together with phosphorus and magnesium. Excess phosphorus could impair calcium absorption. They have partnered some cramping when there is deficit of this mineral. Magnesium can improve calcium absorption. The calcium deficiencies force to break the skeletal system for these minerals.

Phosphore: Participates with calcium is in the maintenance of bones and teeth. Also in almost all metabolic processes such as energy. Cells use to store and transport energy by adenosine triphosphate (ATP). Involved in DNA and in regulating blood PH. The proportion of calcium and phosphorus in the body affects such that the excess or deficit of one affects the other's absorption.

Potassium (Kalium): Balances the water content of the cells and re-moving excess movement of the body. PH and maintains along with sodium, regulates the amount and normal distribution of water. Involved in the construction of proteins. Conducts nerve impulses to muscles and keeps the heart rate. Its deficit could lead to fluid retention and hypertension in addition to cramps from dehydration. It is excreted along with sodium through sweat.

Sulfur: It is composed of some amino acids such as methionine, cystine and cysteine (involved in the configuration of the protein molecules). If he can not form taurine, very important for the muscles. Essential for protein synthesis and formation of various structures such as skin, cartilage, collagen, tendons, keratin and creatinine.

Remember the importance of hydration in your daily routine and more importance if possible while doing sport. An adult requires 2-3 liters of water a day, apart from foods that may also have considerable amounts (more accurately 33.33 milliliters of water per kilo of body weight) to maintain the water balance because it is quite lost in the urine, feces, lungs (exhaled air) and skin (perspiration and sweating). Hence the importance of drinking water because it performs different functions in the body and one of them is the regulation of body temperature. Therefore rehydration with slightly cold water is effective for this principle during activities significant heat. Such is the importance of hydration than sodium, chlorine and potassium could not exercise their vital functions and involved in the generation of electrical impulses, muscle contraction (including the heart), and its functions euhydration (levels normal water through the homoestática renal function), osmolarity (control and evacuation of different solutes) and stimulation of the gland pituitary (preceded by the hypothalamus and releases the antidiuretic hormone (ADH) in the blood. This hormone encourages kidneys to increase water absorption and blood again.

In definitive, water in itself will be more than enough to restore normal levels of electrolytes in your body. Still in very prolonged workouts may be useful solutions of carbohydrates and some minerals. See then your assessment with a specialist.

MICROMINERALS

They are also called as trace elements are so called because they are essential but in very small quantities (less than 100 mg / kg DM). Essential for the normal functioning of almost all biochemical processes in the body.

Besides these nutrients they are part of many enzymes and coordinate a number of biological processes.

Zinc: Absorption increases with the animal, histidine and methionine organic protein and citric acid. It promotes growth and helps improve natural testosterone levels. It contributes as healing of tissues. Increases antioxidant function of vitamin A. (Too much calcium can interfere with the absorption of zinc and copper and iron complementary).

Selenium: Antioxidant and anticarcinogenic. It contributes to detoxify the body from heavy metals storage such as mercury and cadmium. Increases the effectiveness of vitamin
E. Involved in nerve and cardiac system.

Chrome: In picolinate supplement helps regulate blood glucose because it promotes the release of insulin. Involved in the metabolism of macronutrients and with iron, helps transport proteins in the body.

Iron: Involved in the proper functioning of respiration and oxygen transport and the blood system. It combines with proteins to form hemoglobin (red blood pigment) and thus able to transport oxygen to tissues. Strengthens the quality of blood and increases resistance to stress and fatigue and different conditions. Its deficit is related to different anemias and menstruation. Their requirements are higher in periods of pregnancy and lactation.

Copper: Involved in iron metabolism and the formation of erythrocytes (red blood cells). brain and nervous system tissue healing besides giving flexibility to the arteries, intervening in libido and circulation.

Iodo: Involved in thyroid hormones, growth and metabolic regulation.

Manganese: It is found in liver, bones, pituitary gland, kidneys and pancreas. Activates various enzymes and other minerals such as vitamin E and participates in a large number of organic reactions. It is a powerful antioxidant. Involved in the degradation of carbohydrates and fatty acids metabolism.

Regulates blood glucose and intervene in bone density with calcium and vitamin D. Also in the formation of mucopolysaccharides (carbohydrate structures) that comprise cartilage (connective tissue).

FOODS RICH IN MINERALS

What is coming now are a few foods where you can find the richness of various minerals to improve your eating plan.

Calcium: Seaweed, dairy products, sardines, sesame seeds, almonds, spinach, manchego cheese, scampi, prawns, shrimp, nuts and vegetables give us a good dose of this mineral. (Carefully document on coral calcium as it is used for alkalizing, ie increasing body and reducing acidity PH exercise).

Hill: Egg yolk, soybeans, cabbages, chickpeas, lentils, cauliflowers, peanuts, grapes.

Sulfur: Protein-rich foods such as meat, seafood, cheese, vegetables and nuts. (Apart from their functions for the skin and joints, it is interesting to study its intervention in diabetes because it stimulates the production of insulin which is necessary for prevention).

Chrome: Apples, walnuts, barley, broccoli.

Magnesium: Bran, pumpkin seeds and watermelon, cocoa powder, linseed, sesame, walnuts, sunflower seeds, almonds and cashews, millet, rice, wheat and whole oats, soy beans, spinach, broccoli, herbs and spices, avocado, cabbage . (Important to keep the appropriate balance between the magnesium, calcium, vitamin K2, and vitamin D. These four nutrients work together synergistically).

Phosphore: whole grains, meat, soy, fish, walnuts, almonds, hazelnuts, peanuts, beans (beans, beans, beans), products and milk derivatives.

Potassium: Chard, custard apples, potatoes, cabbage, Brussels sprouts, avocado, spinach, bananas. Study your doctor this mineral and involved in the fluid retention, blood pressure and heart rate.

Sodium: Low in sodium are fruits, vegetables, grains, legumes and seeds, on the other hand are high in sodium sausages, fi ambres cured, pickled, canned, prepared foods and salt. (Interestingly in combination with potassium to control moisture balance).

Iron: red meat, seafood, liver, black pudding, sesame nuts, green leafy vegetables, soy, legumes, seaweed, spinach and whole grain products.

Zinc: Oysters, clams, liver, brewer's yeast, meat, sesame and pumpkin seeds, almonds and oats.

Selenium: Oats, walnuts, pumpkin seeds, mushrooms, beans, brewer's yeast.

Fluorine: Salmon, cod, mackerel, pork liver, wheat germ, nuts.

Iodo: Himalayan salt, seaweed, blueberries, strawberries, dairy products, potatoes.

Manganese: almonds, whole grains, tea, avocado.

Copper: Organ meats, red meat, seafood, nuts, cocoa, oats, barley, wheat and other whole grains.

Do not settle, remember that above "good", can be "better". It is important to look down to be grateful for the better situation in which you find yourself, but also looks up, where wealth and success of those people who have achieved success in any area of your life.
Learn, let yourself be impregnated by that mentality, you do checkpoint, incomódate, Push yourself more each day yourself so you can go for what you deserve and I'll see getting it.

4. PROTECTION OF THE JOINTS AND AID IN THE REGENERATION OF THE CARTILAGE

Joint pain can make it difficult in some ways their movements and their athletic performance (even in the most basic everyday tasks). The good news is that apart from getting in the hands of professionals have at their disposal a number of supplements that can bene fi ciarle to ease pain and speed recovery of your joints and presented below.

Glucosamine: (500-1500 mg daily based body composition). Numerous studies on this substance (composed of the combination of glucose and glutamine amino from molecule). Ask in supplement form because it is used by our bodies to contribute in helping tendons, ligaments and other connective tissue problems and improve rheumatoid arthritis. Check with your doctor.

Chondroitin: It is often marketed primarily as chondroitin sulfate. This component is part of a large protein molecule called (proteoglycan) providing cartilage elasticity, this is obtained from different species both marine and terrestrial (shark cartilage, cow ...) and also synthesized in our body. Studies to treat osteoarthritis in horses and dogs for many years have brought that also intend to transfer to humans. Study the benefits in terms of points of joint pain, cartilage degradation, arthritis, gout, osteoporosis and heart functions (500-1200 mg are usually standardized jacks). Talk to your healthcare.

MSM: Methylsulfonylmethane is better known every day due to its properties to relieve joint pain. See their benefits as this natural sulfur compound to the body is an essential part of metabolism supporting collagen formation and intervention in the production of essential amino acids. Often it used for acne, tendinitis, arthritis, bursitis, osteoarthritis, fi bromialgias, cystitis, ulceration, digestive problems, hair, nails and fragile skin, intestinal parasites as well as muscle aches and cramps. (Doses ranging from 50 mg / kg for muscle pain in general and from 1.5 to 6 grams of MSM per day in 3 doses for up to 12 weeks. Some studies show that for 60 days combination with boswellic acid, hydrolyzed collagen, lipase, vitamin C, curcumin and bromelain from pineapple rely on their functions (there are also combos sold in a 3: 2: 2 or 3: 2: 1 of glucosamine, chondroitin and MSM).. Seek advice also with your specialist.

Shark cartilage: It is also used for arthritis, muscle pain, including psoriasis and wound healing, damage to the retina due to diabetes and for bowel inflammation. It is rich in glucosamine. Its content is nothing special about any other animal cartilage. Be sure to follow the relevant product instructions and consult your pharmacist, doctor.

L-methionine: We have included this essential amino acid here because it is important for the formation of cartilage substance sulfur content. In combination with B vitamins, it may form almost all sulfur containing compounds. And by this methionine is particularly important for the following three cases may reduce inflammation, can soothe and stimulate the formation of cartilage cells.

L-cysteine: This nonessential amino acid can also bene fi ciarle in pain and inflammation of joints.

Histidine: Besides being used to improve digestion can support on tissue healing. This nonessential amino acid is usually combined with other supplements to treat rheumatoid arthritis and joint pain.

Proline: Among the many features of this amino acid it is not essential to intervene in the texture of the skin and collagen production through the aging process. Aid in healing cartilage and strengthening of joints, tendons and heart muscles. There are studies that can increase its effectiveness through the use of vitamin B3, C, lysine, serine, threonine, ornithine and glutamine.

Omega 3: Alpha-linoleic (Omega 3) fatty acids bene fi cardiovascular system, improve brain and eye immunity.

Clinical studies indicate that a steady intake of these fatty acids support the reduction of LDL cholesterol and triglycerides. Normally in most European diets (except in some countries) there is a high intake of omega 6 with respect to 3. So you should analyze the benefits of including this latest diet plan regularly as it also intervenes in blood flow and the effects antiin joint fl amatory very suitable in case of arthritis and other rheumatic problems. The dose ranges from 1-3 grams per day, even from 500mg daily and can appreciate its benefits. Sure to select either the source of omega 3 feeds (eg salmon or cod is preferable to other substitutes) and% EPA / DHA complement. EPA (eicosapentaenoic acid) and DHA (docosahexaenoic acid) are two essential polyunsaturated fatty acids omega-3 series and alpha-linolenic coming acid (ALA). Despite being necessary for life, our body is unable to synthesize them and we need an external consumption. So be sure to eat good levels. Consult your specialist.

Conjugated linoleic acid: With respect to (CLA), research is finding that has a wide range of important biological effects both reduce cholesterol, triglycerides and stimulate body fat loss. CLA inhibits enzyme activity Lipoprotein Lipase enzyme that breaks down fat particles in the blood so that they can be absorbed by adipocytes (fat cells) for storage. Therefore, CLA may help you avoid deposition and accumulation of fat in the body and improves blood flow directly involved in the disinflinflammation of the joints. 1-3 grams per day according to body weight. Carefully document further.

MCT oil (Medium Chain Triglycerides): Appear again in this chapter because they increase the presence of ketones which prevent muscle breakdown. Source of calories characterized by a rapid and complete oxidation plus free fatty deposits. Since fatty acid medium chain (MCFA) do not require the aid of carnitine, they are oxidized immediately as energy, while glucose (MCT oil does not travel through the lymphatic system other oils). This use has a preserving effect of glucose and helps glycogen stores last longer. The more lasting glucídicas these reserves can train longer before fatiguing. Since the MCT oil is fully oxidized, it can not be deposited as fat. (It's immediate energy, but with the benefit that it provides twice as many calories), which the body can burn more calories intensely without their glycogen stores are depleted, delaying fatigue and fatigue. Take advice on using this supplement, your level of triglycerides and overall heart health.

Alpha lipoic acid (ALA): Among its various studies highlight the contribution as an antioxidant. It can help you clean up the toxic substances from your liver as it helps in the efficiency of vitamins C and E. Its consumption appears to increase levels of glutathione (a powerful antioxidant produced by the body through amino acids). Also it involved the pancreas to release insulin after training to replenish glycogen stores. It is often used as a supplement One dose after training.

In the market also has supplements hydrolyzed collagen and hyaluronic acid rich in proline, glycine and hydroxyproline (even enriched with vitamins and some coenzymes) which could induce some improvements in certain connective tissues besides levels of elastin.

**There are elderly people
aged 25 and younger than
75.
It's not your age,
it's what you're done!**

5. MUSCLE RELAXANTS AND ANTIDEPRESSANTS, CENTRAL NERVOUS SYSTEM INHIBITORS AND GROWTH HORMONE PRECURSORS

I am fully convinced that it is expanding its information regarding the existence of certain aids that can contribute their joints and bone health. Despite being better informed always remember congruence analyze each add both components, origin, dosification interactions and their seal of quality. We must learn to differentiate between "quantity" of the product and its "purity" that often do not go hand in hand. Explore with more professional if necessary.

Among many in the market below shows some add-ons that could act as relaxing the central nervous system and could contribute you with better sleep and muscle repair.

Melatonin: 1 to 3 milligrams per day according to weight and physical condition (before bedtime). This supplement could maximize hormone produced by the pineal gland regulating the sleep cycle. Check with your doctor.

GABA (gamma amino butyric acid): 50-250 milligrams or spread over several shots before bedtime. This is the main brain inhibitory neurotransmitter acting on the pituitary gland. It helps induce relaxation and sleep (where the excitation of the brain is balanced with inhibition). Acting in reducing neuronal activity, generating a calm and relaxed state of the central nervous system. GABA also can be synthesized by the amino acid glutamine. Vitamin B6, glycine and taurine increase absorption. Numerous studies have been used successfully in the field of hyperexcitability, insomnia, anxiety and depression. Growth hormone is synthesized in anterior regions of the gland pituitary and it is released in gradually throughout the day, which last a short time and are used as are secreted by the gland. Different studies involving HGH levels detected after ingesting high form GABA, (especially in rest periods). The therapeutic dose ranges from 50-250 milligrams or spread over several shots before bedtime.

L-tryptophan: Precursor of serotonin and melatonin (affecting mood and brain activity). This essential amino acid in supplement form can help by relaxing the central nervous system and induce sleep. Their contribution in the production of hydrochloric acid can improve digestion. Studies reveal that may have increased levels of somatotropin (growth hormone) allowing gain more lean muscle mass and increasing the strength. You can also contribute by foods such as meat, eggs, bananas and milk.

Tyrosine: It is also often see added in pre-workout supplements for its stimulation of adrenaline and dopamine. This nonessential amino acid enhances the activity and mental concentration, in fl owing in the central nervous system against anxiety and stress. Mediates the release of growth hormone which could lead to increases in muscle mass when a plan is suitable.

Alpha-GPC (L-alpha glycerylphosphorylcholine): Complement acetylcholine precursor. This metabolite phospholipid is concentrated in neuronal membranes. Alpha-GPC hill fast delivery to the brain through the cerebral blood-brain barrier and inducing higher levels of choline in the brain. That is to say, is a natural precursor physiological acetylcholine, a neurotransmitter involved in memory and other cognitive functions. (There are even potential findings to improve Alzheimer). Studies show increases in growth hormone recording increased fat oxidation when obtaining energy for exercise. Consult your specialist about this natural supplement hill.

External circumstances often can not control, but the
problem is not the pro-
blem, it's your choice, it's
your decision it's your attitude toward what happens
what you will win!

6. IMPROVEMENTS FOR DIGESTION AND ABSORPTION OF NUTRIENTS

Throughout this book I have guidance on the importance of protein synthesis, maintaining good levels of nitrogen regularly in the body (not just the increase in muscle mass if your goal is to improve their image but also for the correct functioning of the organs of your body). We have also studied how you can increase muscle anabolism and recovery thanks to supplements to reduce ammonia, acidity and byproducts generated by physical effort with your eating plan. I've driven it has to meet the needs in macro and important trace minerals your body needs in addition to the proper administration of vitamins, distinguishing water-soluble (those excess are rapidly expelled by the body) and fat soluble (taking more caution in because your intake is stored in the body for various time). He has also done a great learning about some key components that can help (by a fi planned caloric cit) in better utilization of body fat in your goal of getting a body more than fi nest and slender or after a while by volume, if only your goal is to recover your weight battle! I am glad that your mindset is expanding to open the range to new formulas and new components to help fight joint pain and accelerate bone healing.

Will agree there is to know to make good decisions for the future regardless of our age and one of them is taking care of our health, do not you think?

We have target with a few components that can contribute to your rest and relaxation of the central nervous system.

Both strength training programs to programs that need hypertrophy download times and longer recovery.

Some of these substances are secreted properly by the body so their complementarity could be a great boost at this time of the day to day your mind is too active for taking to bed projects, agitation, pressure or circumstances that leave him sleep.

Remember, your goals and your dreams are very important but needs a good rest at night to get up and go with attitude recovered to the next project. Their happiness is not negotiable.

What comes next is very important, even something that many do not know and can contribute you a much needed pillar in the assimilation of your eating plan, ulcers, heartburn, indigestion, irritable colon and stomach different circumstances. Because not only it has to consider what you eat but what is absorbed, I present a list of some digestive enzymes you can get from food but also in higher doses in supplement form. Digestive enzymes are basically produced by different organisms of our body, break the polymers are present in food in much smaller molecules (such as proteins, fats and carbohydrates) so they can be absorbed more easily. Consult your specialist these benefits and the potential to improve food intolerances.

Ptyalin (salivary amylase): This over there in the saliva acts on starch digestion starting at the mouth decomposing mono- and disaccharides.

Amylase: It acts on starches providing glucose. It is produced in the stomach and pancreas.

Pepsin: Secreted by glands in the stomach and is involved in the breakdown of proteins hidrolizándolas chains, ie, separating them into smaller peptides and amino acids.

Lipase: It is produced in the pancreas and is responsible for the degrading them cleave fats glycerine and fatty acids.

Lactase: It occurs in the small intestine (production decreases with growth) and is responsible for digesting lactose into glucose and galactose.

Protease: These enzymes are secreted by the stomach, pancreas and small intestine. They are responsible for breaking the bonds of proteins into peptides and amino acids so that they can be better absorbed.

We can also find these enzymes in the market along with the betaine (and named in the first block ons stimulate protein synthesis). A near derivative hill several studies with positive results in benefits to the synthesis of creatine, stabilization of cellular water balance and protein synthesis, regulation of excess homocysteine (product resulting from the digestion of meat, milk and fish), liver and cardiovascular functions in addition to supporting the intervention of hydrochloric acid in the stomach for better digestion. Check with your specialist to include betaine in your eating plan.

You can also find it on sources like whole wheat bread, buckwheat (very good in vitamins and minerals), rice, oats, quinoa and barley. In vegetables such as beets and spinach, (in fact much competitors use beet root powder before races and workouts because it helps in resistance). Germinated sprouts or alfalfa and soybeans are also rich sources of betaine.

You see, you have many failures in life does not make
you a failure. You're bigger
and can more things than
you think!

SECOND PART

7. PHYTOTHERAPY: THE USE OF PLANTS AND PLANT SUBSTANCES FOR SPORT

By now you will have a better idea of how important it is for our bodies learn to digest food properly to use those nutrients in different
body functions.

Now the good comes, because what is going to start reading below is
the second large block of this book and corresponding to the use of
the active principles of plants and other genres in sports and in health
care . I have divided into different objectives but they all relacionaos
using natural therapies to improve, alleviate or help prevent various
symptoms.

When you finish reading this large block will have a broader view of
their use and contribute to their personal welfare. You will agree with
me that to have a better future we must learn to tell the best decisions
for you?

Mistakes are a source of progress. If you do not make mistakes and not learn if you do not learn no improvements. Take failure as a school and not a burden.

8. ANABOLIC PRINCIPLES OF PLANTS

These are different studies that contribute to anabolism, responsible for the manufacture of body tissues and cellular components and thus could help in muscle development with your exercise and eating plan.

Tribulus terrestris: Is usually taken it encapsulated (due to its strong flavor), divided into several shots and always with food (one before physical activity). This tropical species of vine that grows in sandy soil throughout India, Pakistan, Sri Lanka and northern Australia is known to be a precursor help in increasing testosterone levels. The active components of Tribulus extract are saponins (involved in follicle stimulating hormone (FSH) which is synthesized by the pituitary gland for the proper functioning of the ovaries and testes).

There are numerous studies on increased libido and improved sexual activity in both men and women. If used as a complement note product quality observing concentrations of saponins in the package. See more about this plant.

Fenugreek (Fenugreek): This extract is often marketed in capsules that are taken before meals. Very digestive, appetite stimulant and anabolic. This annual plant cultivated for some time in Asia, particularly in India and China have different studies on reducing blood sugar and cholesterol thanks to its high flavonoid content. Study their different components as it is very rich in fiber, restorative and used to treat anemias.

Maca: It is often marketed powder but consumed raw or cooked. It is native tuber from the Andes in Peru has been used for a long time for its analog and restorative properties. Widely rich in vitamins and minerals acts directly on the nervous system by strengthening the immune system, increasing energy levels and improving overall physical and mental results. Carefully document more about this plant.

Muira puama: This shrub native to the Amazon rainforest in Brazil has studies on libido and sexual function and is considered among the main natural aphrodisiacs in the world.

Yohimbine: The bark comes from a tree native to certain West African countries (Cameroon, Congo, Nigeria). It has been used for many years to increase libido and improve impotence. It is often used in various sports supplements as it helps in vasodilatation and accelerates the heart rate.

Tongkat ali (Eurycoma longifolia): Tree slender trunk rainforest. Tongkat or "cane Ali" is a plant native to Malaysia, lower Burma, Thailand and Indonesia. It is often used as a supplement for its properties to reduce fatigue, increase energy and libido. Different studies have in increasing sperm and increased testosterone levels.

Sarsaparilla (Smilax aspera or Moorish bush): Besides being a very usual bush as a natural remedy to combat skin impurities also it has many androgenic and anabolic properties in fl owing in muscular strength and endurance. Although the fruits have some toxicity, used phytotherapy root (powder or crushed) as it is very rich in choline and mineral salts. It tends to favor the elimination of excess uric acid, purify the blood in addition to cleaning the bladder and kidneys.

Nettle: This is one of the plants that has more medicinal uses. Nettle has numerous studies on testosterone also increases root extract used for prostate health. (The testosterone circulating in the blood is carried by a class of proteins such as SHBG (betaglobulin). Nettle extract favors the release of this protein SHBG, and be free facilitates anabolic processes. Among other properties has high power diuretic therefore it helps eliminate ammonia in urine, stones, gout, etc. deflating loves the prostate is rich in iron uy, improves blood circulation and reduces blood sugar levels.

Goat Weed (Yin Yang Huo): This herb peculiar name is considered by the Chinese to raise the libido and erectile function in men. The plant has been used for a long time to restore sexual passion and dispel fatigue. In botanical medicine in China and Japan it is used for disorders of the kidneys, and joints. Usually it sold mixed with other plants such as maca, muira puama, tongkat ali and ginseng to enhance its effects.

Rhodiola rosea: This traditional plant in Eastern Europe and Asia has a reputation for stimulating the nervous system, libido and combat stress.

Increases the resistance to stress and improve recovery after intense muscular exercise. Its properties allow reducing the concentration of various stress-induced metabolites in the body, particularly the increasing mental fatigue. It has different studies in improving sexual function and bioavailable increases serotonin (a chemical found in the brain that regulates sleep cycle). See more about the benefits of this plant.

Chlorella: This freshwater microalgae has properties similar to spirulina. It is a source of high biological value proteins, amino acids, minerals, vitamins and omega fatty acids. It may contain up to four times chlorophyll (natural disinfectant) spirulina. It is very rich in vitamin C. The alga has a protein content of about 65 grams per hundred and contains all the essential amino acids. Some of its properties because these amino acids are strengthening the immune system, acceleration of wound healing, lesions and ulcers, protection against toxic pollutants, liver detoxification and blood, stimulation of cell growth and regulation, protection the effects of radiation. It is also very rich in lutein (natural pigment that protects the eyes from cataract formation). Usually from marketing as dried product powder, capsules or coated tablets. Check with your specialist.

Oats: This herb is rich in vitamins (B1, B2, B3, B6 and E), minerals (calcium, zinc, copper, phosphorus, iron, magnesium, potassium), protein and fat. Indeed it is one of the cereal with a higher proportion of vegetable fat, about half are unsaturated fats and linoleic acid. It also contains a good amount of fibers that contribute to good intestinal and stomach functioning. Constant use appears to reduce LDL cholesterol and triglycerides and increases good cholesterol (HDL). Possessing slowly absorbed carbohydrates is ideal for release energy steadily and retain the feeling of hunger. It has several benefits such as relieving mild symptoms of mental stress and to aid sleep. Externally to treat inflammations in fl mild skin, such as sunburn, and to accelerate healing of minor wounds. Also interesting studies regarding the use of oats and diabetes.

Quinoa: Also called "mother grain". This interesting cereal had been consumed by the Aztecs and the Incas dating from 5,000 BC It contains all eight essential amino acids among many others (in fact it is used by NASA for foods for astronauts because of its high biological quality). Rich in minerals (calcium, iron, magnesium) and vitamins (C, E, B1, B2, niacin) and fiber.

Its low glycemic level makes it interesting to control cholesterol levels. Its composition does not contain gluten naturally. It is very interesting for athletes because they are high in protein to help muscle and recover from intense workouts. Usually it cooked before being washed to remove the bitter taste produced by saponins.

Chia (Salvia hispanic): Chia seeds noted for their good phosphorus content, magnesium, calcium, potassium, iron plus B vitamins emphasize its high content of fiber. These hydrophilic properties enable the seed to absorb water up to twelve times its own weight, which causes the body extend its state of hydration and consequently the electrolyte balance.

Cinnamon (Cinnamomum verum): Normally used as a seasoning in cooking, cinnamon is a powerful antioxidant and vasodilator. It is highly digestive besides having aphrodisiac properties. With regard to the exercise, when cinnamon is consumed with creatine and simple carbohydrates seems to get further increase the insulin spike making the nutrients come better in muscle cells, ie, assists in the process of transporting glucose from the bloodstream to inside muscle cells where it can be used as energy. Cinnamon mimics insulin and helps reduce cholesterol as well be antiviral. Many athletes include in their breakfasts and food in general.

Ginger (Zingiber of fi cinale): Studies have its stimulant for growth hormone and sex drive properties. It is considered an aphrodisiac because ca fluidifying blood and its content in essential oils and amino acids. This interesting rich in antioxidants and flavor characteristic spicy and medicinal plant brings different benefits in improving diabetes, osteoarthritis, respiratory tract, dizziness, rheumatism and menstrual cramps, flu, colds and migraines.

Highly digestive infusion is usually combined with cinnamon, honey, royal jelly or propolis. Ginger has numerous studies on weight loss and vascularity when combined with a good diet plan and exercise.

Spirulina (Arthrospira): With a history of more than 3500 million years this first life of microalgae is one of the most natural foods rich in vitamins, minerals, amino acids and phytonutrients. About half of the protein content is also is rich in essential fatty acids and rich in potassium, sodium, manganese and iron (among other minerals). It's interesting to athletes who want to add it to your multivitamin and multimineral a 100% natural. Usually it indicated in athletes, children, pregnancy and periods of great physical or intellectual activity but consult with your specialist.

Polypody (Polypodium vulgare): It is medicinal plant grows naturally in most of Europe. This fern can have different benefits to increase muscle mass, strength and endurance. It is often used to improve anemia, fatigue, blood purification, bile and liver disorders.

Amaranth: This native grain center of North America (Mexico and Guatemala) and South America (Peru and Ecuador) has expanded worldwide. The Incas called it "Amaranth" (Little Giant), the Aztecs knew him as "huautli" and Mayans called it "xtes" who used it as a high-yielding crop. This grain is gluten free and compared to other grains is quite high in protein, calcium, iron, phosphorus and carotenoids. It has about 70% of unsaturated fatty acids, including linoleic acid which makes it interesting for good cardiovascular and brain function.

During your adventure you better get used to rejection because maybe the word "yes" do not listen very often. Some do not believe in you, and you ignore hesitate but good courage, push yourself to yourself, learn, give more than anyone works harder than anyone could expect. Do it for you, knowing that you are creating the best version of yourself. If you fall, get up, take every opportunity as if your life depended on it, because some are waiting for you to give up, to not fall, but it's not your fault their lack of commitment, do not be dis-tracted until you get your objectives, working in you, focus, grow, develop your skills and get your wins. Fuck you for all you deserve!

9. STIMULANTS, ADAPTOGENS AND COMPONENTS TO REDUCE FATIGUE AND INCREASE ENERGY

After classifying plants and comment anabolic and invigorating properties will show below some stimulating plants that can bene fi ciarle in that extra push to increase its vitality. Some of these plants could be included in more than one classification as they meet and help the body in multiple roles, if however the cataloged in this way have a preponderance and uses which will be discussed below. Always use caution with their personal interactions (if any) and check with your specialist before any decision.

Panax Ginseng: This species is grown in China and Korea and there are many different varieties. It is classified as a stimulant by its concentration in ginsenosides and adaptogenic properties, that is, to increase the vitality and physical states of fatigue, increase concentration and regulating blood sugar levels. Caution should be exercised, overuse could give palpitations, insomnia or irritability like most stimulants.

Eleutherococcus: Also known as Siberian ginseng. For states of physical, mental fatigue and exhaustion. Increased resistance to different physical stressors, improving psychomotor, physical ability and cognitive function. Unlike Panax Ginseng contains saponins, ginsenosides or panaxosides, but if it contains eleuthero, which has been traditionally used to promote longevity and immune system.

American ginseng (Panax quinquefolium): This species of ginseng contains ginsenosides as if panax, which may have adaptogenic and calming effects on the body. You can bene fi ciarle to reduce mental fatigue, increase vitality, improve digestion and other properties similar to Korean ginseng.

Shiitake mushrooms (Lentinulaedodes), Maitake (Grifola frondosa) or the famous Reishi (Ganodermalucidum): These three medicinal mushrooms have interesting active compounds, particularly polysaccharides, mainly β-glucans, (studied for different conditions and modulate gene expression in different types of cancer). Very rich in protein, vitamins and minerals (iron, phosphorus, selenium, potassium, zinc, manganese, copper and even germanium, the latter studied in the prevention of tumor processes). These fungi besides being adaptogens (increase vitality and combat fatigue) could bene fi ciarle to lower cholesterol and blood sugar. Study more about it.

Guarana (guarana): This plant from the Amazon is a potent alkaloid rich in tannins, saponins and fl avonoles. Stimulating metabolism is accelerating with a mild diuretic effect. It has high doses of caffeine naturally teo lina fi, theobromine and guaranine. It is absorbed more slowly than coffee, and there is much nervousness. Rich in antioxidants, antiviral and analgesic.

Coffee (coffee tree): With multiple functions for the body, this shrub native to Ethiopia would be introduced to Arabia, from where it would spread through the rest of the world. Marketed from your own drink even in different formats going ons sports coffee is a powerful stimulant alkaloid used to reduce fatigue and increase vitality. When an eating plan takes into deficit calorie and proper training could influence with fat loss because it speeds up metabolism. A portion also can be used as thermogenic. Consult your specialist about different interactions such as arrhythmias, insomnia and various cardiovascular and brain functions to be careful in its administration.

Yerba mate (Ilex paraguariensis): Native to Paraguay and common in the cuisine of Argentina, southern Brazil, Uruguay, Bolivia and Chile and other countries is a powerful source of xanthines (caffeine, theobromine, theophylline), compounds that stimulate the central nervous system by increasing energy levels and concentration. It is a powerful antioxidant (for its high content of polyphenols). It helps maintain healthy blood. It stimulates the production of cortisone and is very diuretic. Studies show that could influence consumption in lowering cholesterol (LDL) and triglycerides.

Kola nut (Cola acuminata): Native to tropical Africa and popularized in the eighties by one of the leading brands of soft drinks in the world is also a powerful stimulant of the central nervous system. Rich in xanthine, (Caffeine), plus tannins (catechol, epicatecol, fl obafenos and potassium salts). It is often combined with guarana, yerba mate and other species to fight fatigue and asthenia. It is softer than tea. Cardiotonic and diuretic.

Or you're too young to begin
or you're too old to fulfill
your goals, no heavier
Shackle to think of a number rather than in your
dreams.

10. PROPERTIES FOR SUPPORT IN THE LOSS OF FAT

All these species we have seen in the previous section are also precursors to fat loss because they are indirectly accelerating metabolism when accompanied by a calorie de fi cit. Even so, this chapter will add some more bene fi ciarle to get a better shape due to its different components.

Garcinia cambogia (HCA): Also called Malabar tamarind is a shrub that grows mostly south India. Originally from more than 200 species of Asia, Polynesia and Africa. This rich thermogenic HCA (Hydroxycitric Acid) is the active ingredient of thousands of nutritional supplements to enhance fat loss, reducing appetite and weight loss. This is because it limits the transformation of carbohydrates into fat by the inhibition of an enzyme called ATP citrate lyase that converts citrate, fatty acids and cholesterol first step fat synthesis. HCA produces satiety by stimulating the liver gluco-receptor. This is achieved because on one hand reduces the production of fats and other increases production of glycogen. You can get it in health food stores or specialty stores.

Glucomannan: This fiber is mostly used in supplements to whet the appetite as this gel in contact with the stomach he is able to multiply percent volume thereby reduce hunger and satiate. In the fi nal not only glucomannan but the fi soluble fibers in general can help depending on your eating plan to improve your cholesterol, triglycerides and blood sugar, besides reducing the glycemic index of foods when ingested together.

Fucus: This type of algae from the Atlantic coast and North America are rich in protein, vitamins and minerals. They can stimulate the thyroid and increase metabolism so used as a supplement in capsules or mixed with other fruits and vegetables slimming drinks as it helps regulate the amount of fat in foods by absorbing and removing debris. Rich in fiber so it can reduce heartburn, cholesterol and improve digestion. Outwardly also it used for both skin eczema and ulcers for their bactericidal properties. Consult your specialist and consúmalas a reliable source.

Green tea (Camellia sinensis) and its different varieties: The tea itself is a powerful antioxidant. Numerous compounds have bene fi in leaves such as EGCG (epigallocatechin gallate) and other notable healing substances, including fl uorine, catechins and tannins. High polyphenol (very benefits to the skin and to stabilize blood pressure). Of the four primary polyphenols for example the Green Tea, the (EGCG) is the most effective. Even this powerful antioxidant has been used as preventive contributions for cancer. It is very thermogenic and diuretic controlling blood sugar levels. Among other varieties has the oolong tea "Wu long" (blue tea) more traditional, semi-fermented, or black tea (oxidized greater), both help cardiovascular functions. He White tea It is perhaps the richest in antioxidants (even more than green) and then can also find the Red tea "Pur-erh" widely used to reduce blood fat levels and help digestion. It is what the variety of tea can be used as infusion (each tea requires a different temperature), capsules (if you want to bring a record), include them as cold drinks in your bottle of training or add them in household water and take them over all day for your transfers. Also often accompanied by lemon and other citrus.

WHAT ARE FEELING YOUR BODY REGARDING YOUR WAY OF LIFE?

It is probably something you already know but your habits are very important and your quality of life as well. Not only is fat loss or a better body, gee! It is your continuous thoughts, mind and spirit.

Ask yourself, "What am having faith and how to visualize the day? Do I see a gray future using most of the excuses that people use or a promising future because I know that everything depends on me?. "

Something that I fully agree is that most specialists focus on treating a condition or a disease when this has occurred. But what about all the external conditions that are fueling this anxiety? Maybe it's just a little anxiety, stress, or have crazy head back in your stuff and need fresh air, new experiences and do different things. People often wonder why I get up so early, "7/7" (seven days a week). It is simple, but sometimes I make mistakes and I think not waste my time. You can sleep late and spew doing things fast and all milk or you can get up a few hours before, making the bed, meditate as many successful people do, prepare your cup of tea, read, study, exercise, shower to activate your metabolism and be prepared for the day. I assure you that all the elite fail to do unimaginable things in those early morning hours, The creativity and productivity are infinite!

It may seem a trite phrase but just make retrospection in yourself, devote yourself quality time and analyze yourself so you can improve, believe me almost nobody does, it will reduce your anxiety and results will begin to applaud.

Get your productivity from early to prepare your day, make plans, not simply leave everything to the free will and mental notes, write them! The mind must be as free fi sufficiently so you can think about your next move and get new ideas.

Remember that your thoughts lead your life, too many people are involved in the side effects of negativity and emotional roots that produce stress.

It is therefore important to plan your space for you, daily and weekly. That does not mean you do the bum! For many people feel worse by two things: doing absolutely nothing or want to do everything. It produces the same anxiety one than the other. So free your mind and give yourself space in different activities. One of the many you can do is thank truth when you wake up all you have: from where you sleep, your life, whom you know, you've done ...

Thank and bless everything you do. When you value what you have, you are sending messages of abundance, you attract good and you just start to get more. Your body will be the first to feel these benefits.

And an important point to keep in mind: to prolonged calorie de fi cit hormone levels leptin blood begin to decline, losing thyroid stimulation and slowing metabolism.

This would produce more hunger and appetite (because it is not inhibited as such the production of certain peptides) accompanied by a lower caloric expenditure. It is therefore important that if you are in deficit, raise your calorie plan at certain times to restore leptin levels since this hormone produced by adipocytes and once freed, begins to act on the hypothalamus to control appetite level. Rely on his professional.

There are already too many people doing the same thing in this world, complain. Since when a broken mill approaches the wind? Change your mind! You are not to mourn, you are to sell handkerchiefs.

11. DIURETICS: RELEASE OF FLUID RETENTION, URINARY SYSTEM AND PROSTATE

The accumulation of fluid in the tissues for example in the belly, ankles or wrists could be harmful to health, especially in pregnant women and people with disabilities. The good news is that there are a number of natural diuretics that now discover that regardless of your current situation either athlete or not, you pave the way. This section not only will we present some diuretic plants that can help reduce or prevent fluid retention (dropsy), but also some fruits and vegetables for their interesting properties that can give you an extra conditioning.

Dandelion: Plant growing in the regions of Europe, Asia and North America is very diuretic. With a mild laxative effect. It helps eliminate liver toxicity, improve the function of this and gallbladder. Consumed speeds digestion and the appetite. Source of vitamins and minerals (especially potassium). It is one of the plants that can further increase urine output.

Horse tail: Highly diuretic and remineralizing due to its rich potassium salts, flavonoids and sapon. Its high silica fi jar helps calcium to bones so he could bene fi if osteoporosis. Widely used for fluid retention, kidney stones, urinary tract infections, cystitis, urethritis, inflammation of the bladder or prostate.

Rusco: This medicinal part used and added in many preparations to relieve circulatory disorders is a potent releaser retention of liquids. It has more than ten components diuretics including steroidal saponins, glycolic acid and minerals such as calcium, magnesium or potassium. It can relieve gout problems, inflammation of the veins, varicose veins and cellulite.

Corn: One of the most important in stimulating diuresis, cleanse the kidneys and lower blood pressure resources. Treats cardiac failure and renal science, relieves the kidneys and helps remove gall stones. In addition to poultices, infusions are often made also with the beard of corn to increase the amount of urine and urinary tract clean.

Bearberry (Grape ursi): The leaves of this plant have a high diuretic power. It is a natural antibiotic against infections of the urinary tract: urethritis, pyelitis, cystitis and also for the treatment of kidney stones. Be careful with your contraindications and consult your specialist.

Orthosiphon: It helps eliminate gallstones and kidney (kidney stones). As an infusion, the sheets are indicated orthosiphon to increase diuresis, especially when there are pictures of inflammation and grittiness in the kidneys. Also often it used in treating bacterial infections of the urinary tract.

Pellitory: Highly diuretic because tannins, flavonoids and potassium salts. Used to aid in the boxes cystitis, ureteritis, urethritis, pyelonephritis, oliguria, hyperuricemia, hiperazotemia, reduce uric acid and hypertension besides blood retention. Usually it used as infusion, syrup or extract fluid.

Parsley: Curiously, it is one of the best diuretics helping to prevent the formation of kidney stones among other properties. Feel free to add to your dishes if you have the opportunity to do so.

Pear: This fruit is rich in potassium, magnesium, zinc, vitamin C and arginine. It has considerable power diuretic, increasing urination much. Favors clean uric acid, kidney and gallbladder. It is highly digestible and even very rich in complex sugars can take the diabetics since such sugars are released gradually into the body by a low glycemic index.

Goldenrod: It is used to increase diuresis in fl inflammations and reduce infections and urinary tract stones.

Purslane: Diuretics and very cleansing. It helps to dissolve kidney stones and deflating love the urinary tract. Purslane is commonly used externally as eye drops, to cleanse and soothe irritations.

Vulnerary: As an infusion it is quite cleansing and mild laxative. Externally as fluid is impregnated in gauze to apply on wounds and burns because it helps heal and disinfect.

Fennel: The stems of this plant are very moisturizing. Promote digestion, are diuretics (lower the blood pressure) and are also used as infusion of different forms: as a home collyrium (prevents glaucoma, tired eyes, sties), mouthwashes, (inflammation of the gums) and skin (eczema and burns). It is also rich in alanine (increasing defenses), arginine and histidine. It is also very rich in iron.

American dwarf palm Saw (Saw Palmetto, Sabal, Serenoa repens): Used in Europe, Canada and the United States. Especially for men over 40, saw palmetto extract may be the first line of defense against benign prostate adenoma. Since about 40% of men over 50 years experience benign prostatic hyperplasia (BPH) (enlargement of the prostate that can result in some cases urinary problems and urination). Some studies show that could be as efficacious in the treatment of BPH as prescription drugs but without these adverse effects. In final often it used in cases of prostatitis that saw palmetto prevents testosterone into dihydrotestosterone, or DHT become. That is, the increased levels of DHT is also partly responsible for benign prostatic hyperplasia. Saw palmetto inhibits the activity of estrogen receptors and also raising testosterone levels. For men who do mostly sport and aim to increase muscle mass or just want to have a better silhouette should remember to increase the consumption of good fats such as unsaturated or polyunsaturated fats and reduce saturated. This is very important because fat cells, the enzyme "aromatase" contact begins testosterone biosynthesis by increasing the conversion into estradiol (estrogen). Testosterone produced by the leydig cells in the testes may be affected by decreasing sexual development among other functions. Why saw palmetto American saw has all natural anabolic properties to help grow and strengthen muscles. Check with your specialist.

Pumpkin: For their different properties (in addition to its high zinc content) pumpkin seeds are used to treat micturition problems associated with benign prostatic hyperplasia, irritable bladder and intestinal parasites.

Cherry tree: Rich in tannins and high flavoniods power diuretic cherry can also be used to treat urinary tract infections, excess uric acid, gout, hypertension, edema and overweight accompanied retention.

Strawberry (Strawberry): Diuretic and antirheumatic help eliminate excess uric acid. Favoring low levels of cholesterol, linolenic acid content, vitamin C (more than oranges) and E having. Antiin amatoria and rich in antioxidants fl. In women is also important consumption during pregnancy and nursing mothers because it contains folic acid, potassium and fiber.

They may also be interested gooseberry, celery, alfalfa or watercress because apart from bring you many other benefits are also very diuretic. Its consumption can help prevent or relieve excess uric acid, improve liver function and kidney stones and gall bladder.

Never hang your head in adversity. Put attitude towards what you want and no matter what happens, Fight to get it!

12. IMPROVEMENT OF THE CIRCULATORY SYSTEM AND VASCULARITY

Ginkgo Biloba: Promotes good blood circulation and cerebral functionality, can improve memory and concentration as it contains flavonoids, terpenoids and ginkgoloides which have antioxidant properties. These substances contribute to destroy free radicals that disrupt cell membranes and DNA. Increases transmission neural impulses as indicated and could him away from the associated disorders fi cits blood circulation in the brain along with thromboembolism, arteriosclerosis, stroke, varicose veins and cardiovascular problems.

Since ginkgo improves blood circulation could improve sexual function also could be used with ginseng, maca, tribulus terrestris, or rhodiola rosea to improve its antioxidant and energy capabilities. Carefully document about using this supplement for Alzheimer's, Parkinson's, Down syndrome, arrhythmias, glaucoma, as well as the help of different chemotherapies.

Hawthorn (Hawthorn): Plant from the center of Europe. Also it has vasodilatory properties of arteries and cardiotonic. Flavonoids (quercetin, rutin, vitexin, catechins) together with magnesium, potassium, calcium and the neurotransmitters dopamine and purine adenine minerals are responsible for this property. It helps the heart pump blood better by improving circulation. Also it has a relaxing effect and sedative (nerves and insomnia).

Buckeye: Antin amatorio and recommended for circulatory inadequacy and cerebral venous fl science. Aesculina and aescin rich, two interesting components that have the ability to prevent edema and could increase the resistance of blood vessels. Therefore it is used for circulatory diseases such as heaviness, swelling, pain, varicose veins, cellulite, tingling and night cramps. Rich in vitamin C, quercetin, rutin, flavonoids, tannins and saponins. In men, horse chestnut has also been used for inflammation of the prostate (benign prostatic hyperplasia). Check with your specialist the different properties of horse chestnut.

Vid (common Parra, red vine): The infusion of the leaves are commonly used for the treatment of chronic venous inadequacy science and poor circulation (swelling of the legs, varicose veins, arteriosclerosis, cerebral circulation, hemorrhoids, vaginal bleeding, arteriosclerosis among other conditions). Its leaves are rich in resveratrol, a powerful antioxidant with several benefits for the immune system. Fruit (grapes) are very rich in vitamins, minerals and amino acids. Externally the sap of the vine is also used for boxes conjunctivitis, sties and skin conditions.

Tomato: Studies indicate the antioxidant properties of lycopene (red coloration) Tomato could help prevent many cancers. Lowers cholesterol and lowers blood pressure. Rich in vitamin A, C, potassium and calcium. Also rich in glutathione, an antioxidant that helps to eliminate free radicals. It has amounts of butyric gammaaminoácidos

"GABA" (main inhibitory neurotransmitter in the brain) that stimulates growth hormone and improve sleep quality. Rich in fiber may help in circulatory disorders.

Garlic: It could be perfectly in section of medicinal plants anabolic, or remineralizantes. It helps reduce fat in the bloodstream. Improves circulation in the peripheral arterial vascular disorders (hypertension, arterial disease and thrombosis). By its antimicrobial action (allicin content) is useful for combatting colds and other respiratory tract infections, treatment of hypertension, intestinal parasites, infections of the urinary tract. It is often used in sports for its energizing and antioxidant properties. Externally it indicated in osteoarticular pain and antiseptic applied to the skin.

Onion (Allium cepa): Besides being used in different dishes in gastronomy, you could bene fi ciarle in preventing atherosclerosis by the properties it contains. Also for reducing blood glucose in diabetes I and II. Rich in vitamins A, B, C, sulfur, iron, iodine, potassium and sodium onion could dissolve uric acid (responsible for the disease gout which affects the kidneys and joints), since infection control thanks to sales of soda and potash, which alkalize the blood. (Same taxonomic family that garlic). It could prevent osteoporosis, due to its high content of quercetin avonoide fl. In fi nal consumption of onions in your food plan could favor him to protect the cardiovascular and urinary system in addition to the prostate. Curiously sauces or dressings garlic, onion, olive oil, with added parsley, bay, oregano, red pepper, basil and rosemary makes an interesting combination for their antioxidant, medicinal and energizing properties.

Yucca: Very interesting for its anti-cancer properties for the circulatory system. Used for rheumatoid arthritis (gout, fibromyalgia). It contains resveratrol one flavonoid that fluidifying ca blood (decreases platelet aggregation) and which could help to reduce cholesterol. Its properties make it interesting against arteriosclerosis, angina pectoris and thrombi. It can be used externally for its analgesic and anti-in ammatory to massage battered areas and joint pain fl.

Psyllium (Plantago psyllium): Apart from being interesting to reduce diabetes and prevent the absorption of "bad" LDL cholesterol and prevent gallstones, this species is very rich in fiber (mucilage). So it is an excellent laxative and it can relieve in cases of constipation, pregnancy, dysentery, intestinal peristalsis and irritable bowel syndrome.

Lettuce: Plentiful vitamin A, C, K, B1, B2, B3, magnesium, calcium and potassium. All varieties including Canons have a low caloric intake, which helps in weight control plans and richness in fiber (1-2 grams per hundred). In addition, the consumption of different types such as red leaf, green, romaine, beluga, tudela, butterhead, batavia or iceberg among other favors prevent high blood pressure, kidney pain, stones and renal failure, inflammation of the bladder (cystitis). Improves circulation (atherosclerosis) and release cholesterol (LDL). It also facilitates digestion and protects the stomach. Your home infusion may be as eye drops.

Sugar cane: Nutrients both raw and juiced provide very good properties. Besides its sweetening power, molasses contains calcium, iron, magnesium and potassium. It has a low glycemic index and can help prevent coronary, arterial circulatory risks, liver disorders and hypertension besides improving vitality. Please do not confuse it with sugar "brown" or so-called "sugar cane" because marketing makes these products are marketed as such when in fact it is white table sugar toasted pretending that golden color brown. Get it from sources fi ables because molasses should be quite thick and stick to your fingers.

Raspberry (Rubus idaeus): Rich in fiber and potassium raspberry leaves are used in decoction for all conditions related to skin wounds, eczema, itchy skin or acne. Purifying kidney, liver and blood. In rinse the throat, sore throat and mouth sores. Its fruits are very rich in antioxidants (flavonoids that these both raspberry and different varieties of berries are related to improved memory, cognitive ability and less talk cell aging studies). Raspberries could bene fi ciarle for cardiovascular functions also are rich in vitamin C and lutein (natural pigment of the retina responsible for improving vision).

Apple: Anabolic charged amino acids (glutamine, glycine, lysine, arginine, histidine, serine, tyrosine, methionine, leucine, isoleucine, valine) aspartic acid among others. Highly digestive, Antin fl amatory, combat ulcers and stomach problems, vasodilator, regulates nitrogen. Diuretic and cleansing. Reduces cholesterol and hypertension. Anticancer. It could help you sleep better rich in tryptophan. Lot of malic acid (the sour taste especially green apples) involved in the ATP and Krebs cycle (energy production) as well as detoxifying and bactericide. (Curiously to treat fi bromialgias there benefits using magnesium and malic acid). In addition natural apple juice has great power to blood tonic and diuretic also help dissolve gallstones and kidney.

Mistletoe: Mistletoe berries have numerous antioxidant properties. Carefully document their uses because it can promote to control blood pressure, relieve symptoms of kidney stones and improve circulation. Before consult your specialist.

Primula: Primrose seeds contain mainly omega 3 and omega 6 (linoleic acid and linolenic acid), both fatty acids are essential for our improving circulation and general health agency. The sheets produce a calming effect. Outwardly also often it used in oil format for atopic dermatitis, eczema and acne.

Soy lecithin: Substance formed by Hill (group B vitamins) and fatty acids. It can be found in eggs, liver, legumes, cereals and dandelion. Soy lecithin curiously has emulsifying properties, it fat mixture with water body to support expulsion (interesting against fatty liver disease). Further it provides elasticity to cell membranes to protect them from destruction of free radicals (rich in essential fatty acids omega 3 and 6, phosphorus and potassium). Enables input and output of nutrients within the cells. It could reduce cholesterol, stress and blood clots. It is also rich in phosphatidylserine (as explained in this book), vitamin E and choline. In addition bene fi t to improve memory, alleviate Alzheimer's disease, improve blood circulation by lowering LDL cholesterol and increase vitality.

Beer yeast: Widely used in sports and healthy lifestyles for their energy intake, yeast is an underrated celled fungus that is obtained from the decomposition of gluten malt or barley. But it is a complete source of vitamins (B group) and minerals (potassium, magnesium, iron, copper, zinc, manganese, nickel, silica, chromium ...). It could increase appetite, reduce cholesterol and blood glucose levels. In addition biotin content (B8) makes it interesting for hair, nails and skin. Regulates the function of the thyroid gland and contribute to regenerate the intestinal fl ora.

Celery: Consumption of these buds and their stems stimulate kidney function and help to purify the blood. It is very diuretic and used in different beverages purificant along with other fruits and vegetables. It could regulate cholesterol and blood pressure in addition to heartburn, improve digestion and has anti-inflammatory properties. We favor in cardiovascular function since it is rich in vitamin K, A, C, B, folic acid, fiber and potassium. Try mixing it with other foods and create their own smoothie "detox" (cucumber, lemon juice, apple, pineapple, strawberries or berries, carrots, spinach, pear, orange, algae, etc). They are also very alkaline (pH will increase their body reducing the acidity and fatigue). Make combinations at will and give yourself the opportunity to improve these purificant drinking beverages loaded with vitamins and minerals for example in the morning or after physical activity.

Whole wheat: It reduces cholesterol and can prevent cardiovascular disease. This good carbohydrate source is rich in protein, vitamins (E and B) and minerals (iron, selenium, zinc, potassium, phosphorus, magnesium) addition along with corn, barley, spelled, rye are a very good source fiber improving intestinal transit.

As you might have noticed, there are industries that sell and promote "exclusive" and miracle products announcing that they are the only ones that can lower your "bad" LDL cholesterol, however it has at its disposal a number of opportunities (and many more) as those we have presented and that can help you improve your cardiovascular system very favorably among other functions.

With respect to reduce Cholesterol l (and if it can depending on tolerances, allergies and food plan) also remember to incorporate essential fatty acids such as the avocado, (rich in vitamins D, E, potassium, magnesium, calcium and iron), and you can even find bottled as oil in the supermarket. Or as the sesame (B, minerals and properties antiin ammatory fl) rich in antioxidants, vitamins. The olive (rich in polyunsaturated fatty acids, regulates blood pressure and diabetes in addition to preventing joint pain), or evening primrose oil, (rich in gamma-linolenic acid which contributes to better blood circulation and control of blood pressure).

Another very important point to note regarding your cholesterol and your cardiovascular activity is to stay away completely from the
Trans fat. The problem with this type of unsaturated fat that is saturated by industrial processes. This solidification makes preservative in many foods such as meat, sausages, processed foods, margarines, pastries, chips, crackers, snack ... This type of fat besides being harmful to the body easily skyrocket your LDL cholesterol and triglycerides. That if, on the labels of products like the they will try to sneak because they will not put "trans fats" as such. They seek less harmful names like "industrial fat", "fat obtained by industrial process", "partially hydrogenated oils", "hydrogenated vegetable oil" Watch out for that! It seems that this great discovery to create margarines and butters replace saturated fats is not as good as previously thought. Many in their wrappers put "zero cholesterol" with the aim to captivate the ignorant buyer only to discover on the label are loaded with hydrogenated oils, trans. Even the European Union advised not to consume more than 2% trans fat of total daily calories. Why is that? Anyway, back to our business and with respect to smoothies "detox" I mentioned him earlier could add grated ginger (carefully because it has a strong flavor) because it promotes circulation, flui-

difying cando blood and preventing heart disease. Also instead of "just water" could add infusion chicory, used to regulate blood pressure and deflating love joints plus bactericide. It is rich in amino acids and minerals and is interesting for anemias and increased vitality.

Also, if you can not control the bitter taste of the smoothie, you can add a bit of natural sweetener stevia (monitor its source as there are some preparations with low purity) will also can promote to regulate blood pressure and blood glucose.

Stay away from whiners, troublemaker, pessimistic, lumps of salt, toxic people, ice blocks, critics and other chicks coming that the sky is falling, no matter what you say or do, they will seek a calamity in every opportunity.

13. RELAXANTS AND RE-LEASERS OF MUSCLE TENSION

In this section, we will present a range of species that can help you sleep, relieve anxiety and definitive ease tensions in your body. Usually indicated in times of stress, or before going to sleep. Most of these plants release GABA, one of the substances that will bene fi t and is used by neurons to communicate with each nervous system. The role of GABA is inhibit or reduce neuronal activity so low levels of this neurotransmitter are associated with stress, anxiety, depression, insomnia and schizophrenia.

Valerian: This perennial plant in North America and Europe relaxes muscles and induces deep sleep. It helps produce and release GABA. Its properties make balance the central nervous system acting as an anxiolytic. It is used against anxiety and insomnia could even treat depression, hypertension and relieve rheumatic pains. You can be in different formats.

Hypericum (St. John's Wort): It is considered a natural antidepressant. It might work by preventing reabsorption of serotonin in the brain relieving depression and stress. Also it induces a relaxing sleep. Alleviating migraine as well as certain types of headaches, muscle pain and nerve pain.

Lemon balm (Melissa): This perennial herb of the family Lamiaceae, native to southern Europe is prized for its strong scent of lemon. Its infusion is used as a natural tranquilizer. Melissa has the ability to calm the heart muscle and restore normal heart rhythm so it is interesting to relieve arrhythmias. It is also highly digestive so often used along with lemongrass to help increase the production of bile. Outwardly it helps to soothe the pain (joints, teeth, ears, etc). Because of its analgesic properties can pour into the bath water and stay within it a few minutes for a deep relaxing bath.

Lemongrass: Widespread worldwide and traditionally used for treating mild to moderate depression. It is very digestive and relaxing addition to antitussive and antispasmodic. Rich in antioxidants and fungicide.

Tila: Linden combat insomnia and relaxes. It is used to regenerate the liver as it can stimulate flow and drainage of bile through this, being effective to descongestionarlo. It is vasodilator and analgesic. Mixed with equal parts bearberry could prevent kidney stones.

Orange blossom: White lemon and orange flower. If female species is interesting because its calming effects could help eliminate discomfort caused by nerves, cramps, headaches, dizziness and menstrual discomfort. Involved in the release of GABA.

Birch: Antiin-inflammatory and diuretic. Rich in essential oils and flavonoids such as quercetin, carotene, tannins and vitamin C. It is also an activator of urine and overall body debugger. Birch has the ability to reduce blood pressure in addition to soothe headaches. It is very purifying and may favor to drain the kidneys, urinary tract infections, arthritis, arthritis and rheumatism.

Passiflora incarnata (Passion Flower): Interesting to relieve insomnia, anxiety, migraine and muscle fatigue. It is very calming. It helps to sleep. It helps to release GABA.

Lavender: It is soothing, analgesic, antiseptic and very digestible. Outwardly the fluid has been used for pain of all kinds in addition to wash small cuts, bites or bruises. It can be used in mouthwashes and mouth conditions.

Hop: Often it used in beer for their flavoring properties. It may be interesting for women as it has a high concentration of phytoestrogens fi and can help
the functioning of the female endocrine system. It is also used for anxiety, nervousness and difficulty sleeping. It is very diuretic and could release GABA.

Rooibos: Really it is not a tea but an infusion not because it comes from the camellia sinensis, but a shrub originating in South Africa. Its properties are very similar to the effects of red tea. It is high in fl uoride, calcium and magnesium plus vitamin C is very alkaline (to combat body acidity) and rich in numerous antioxidants (e.g. quercetin) and flavonoid that could help control blood pressure, combat free radicals and purify the body. It helps relieve anxiety and stress the heart muscle. No doubt the infusion of rooibos can bene fi ciarle to improve your overall health status.

Stop worrying about what people think and start to take care of all the wonderful things you have left to do.

14. DIGESTIVE SYSTEM: ULCERS, VARIOUS DISORDERS, INDIGESTION AND GASTROINTESTINAL DETOXIFICATION

As you may have noticed the active principles of plants are very interesting, in fact most they were used for centuries. Thanks to new developments we have been able to extract more information from them and which could often enjoy the benefit and added quality without being exposed to such toxicity and side effects of medications today. What I am trying to say is that apart from ordinary medicines, may also notice that you have other beneficial much more natural alternatives around, so they can be applied as needed.

As proof will read below a list of genres that will help to alleviate many disorders of the digestive tract, as well as detoxify the body, possible prevention of disease and purifying effects.

Aloe vera: This native to Africa and cultivated in many parts of Latin America, USA and the Canary Islands has entered strongly in both the cosmetics industry and care within the agency for its medicinal and antibacterial properties, purifying species.

Internally aloe gel that is transparent gelatinous substance leaving clear if we press a cut sheet is used. Has many components like modin, aloeoleína, aloetina or aloina, which regulate the pH of the stomach and reduce acidity, while enhancing reflux.

It is very digestive and healing, that their enzymes involved in stimulating the body's defenses and plant hormones that promote healing of tissues is due. It is also rich in folic acid, choline, various amino acids and a source of vitamins A, C and E and of group B. Interestingly has emolina, emodin and barbaloina generating substances salicylic acid (an analgesic and antipyretic effect).

Externally applied to the skin to improve its condition and also favor their mucilage, saponins, mucopolysaccharides and mannose phosphates which are involved in the healing, hydrating and disinfected.

Why it could help improve stomach problems, heartburn, ulcers and slow digestion. Keep an eye on all formatting and recourse if the natural plant leaves and open them it is possible to obtain the gel as there are numerous supplements and creams on the market with very little purity and percentage that can not justify its high price. Always consult your specialist.

Or chamomile (chamomile): Ideal for stomach and intestinal symptoms. Soothing tonic and vasodilator. Highly digestible so its content might prevent and relieve gastric ulcers. It is diuretic and antis-pasmodic plus antiinflamatory (in women may help in the premens-trual pain). Benefit eliminate uric acid and protect the liver. Out-wardly very interesting is its infusion of cold form com eyedrops home as well as disinfects and moisturizes for mouthwashes, tootha-ches and other conditions of the mouth. You can also add it to your water during times of physical activity or their meals because their substances favor relaxing the intestinal muscles. It can be mixed with anise as it is highly digestive (gas, heartburn, stomach pain and nerve damage).

Alfalfa: In this case this kind would help contribute to digestion as it contains enzymes to digest extra protein we take in our food plan. Like chamomile or anise bene fi t against stomach ulcers, heartburn and gas. It is also rich in vitamins and minerals.

Ginger: Here again it appears to improve digestion and reduce gastrointestinal problems. Its properties mean that it can bene fi t in cases of dizziness or vertigo because when digested also focus on keeping the tone of intestinal muscles acting as anti-in fl amatory and antispasmodic helping to prevent fading.

Turmeric: Intense flavor and slightly spicy turmeric is an important medicinal plant as it relieves indigestion, irritable bowel problems and has properties
hepatoprotectoras for the liver and the kidneys. It seems that their colagogas properties and coleréticas improve digestion of fats. It is widely used for these liver disorders (cleaning due to alcohol detoxification, fatty liver, cirrhosis, jaundice, hepatitis, inadequacy biliary science, high cholesterol) as well as other intestinal diseases (colitis, irritable bowel syndrome) and in fl ammatory in general. In combination with cayenne pepper and black pepper increases the absorption of curcuminoids, substances that enhance disin fl inflammation of the relevant affected areas. Its antioxidant properties may help prevent certain cancers such as breast, colon, duodenum, or skin.

Mint: It has numerous properties as an expectorant (expulsion of accumulated bronchial secretions) and the digestive and respiratory (cramps, abdominal pain syndrome irritable bowel, dyspepsia, nausea, allergic rhinitis, asthma and muscular pain). It could be combined with fl or elderberry and ginger tea to relieve colds and flu.

Chicory: Their benefits in smoothies "detox" make it very interesting this species. Moreover consumption (if not allergic or intolerant) stimulates the production of gastric juice which promotes digestion and stimulates the production of bile.

Artichoke (Cynara scolymus): Famous in many eating plans and haute cuisine is also noted for its contents cinarina, chemical and lead compound active component of the plant has choleretic properties (activates the production of bile) and colagogas (facilitate the removal of bile). The artichoke is also highly digestible, and like thistle might reduce cholesterol levels relieving liver cells and gall bladder, stimulating the production of bile juices.

Marshmallow (Althaea officinalis of): It has emollient and demulcent properties, relieving irritation of mucous membranes, (bronchitis, asthma and cough) and stomach (gastritis, ulcers and stomach pain). Externally and their properties alleviates eye baths, sprains and skin conditions.

Papaya or "Lechosa" Laden digestive enzymes help produce gastric juice and better digest food. Improves bowel and liver problems. In the digestive enzymes from papaya aid dissolution of fats. Besides these papain, chymopapain, and glicilendopeptidasa caricaina are cysteine protease enzymes containing about 200 amino acids and which are stabilized by three disulfide bridges. In simple words are a potent mixture of proteolytic enzymes and can help the absorption and protein synthesis when consumed together. It   is also anti-in fl amatory, prevents heartburn and stomach ulcers, favoring relief surgeries, edemas and irritation in the intestine.

Cayenne pepper: Interestingly for some have six times more potassium than a banana, is rich in magnesium, calcium, phosphorus, zinc, vitamin A, groups B, C and K. It is also very rich in protein and fiber. Some of the interesting benefits is that it helps to produce stomach acid to digest food better and heal stomach ulcers. Capsaicin cayenne (among other alkaloids) is the substance that produces heat and burning, it stimulates blood circulation, accelerating metabolism and causing the brain to release endorphins (natural opiácidos that increase the sense of well being in the body).

Plum: They are rich in fiber and sorbitol, which help regulate the operation of the system and facilitate digestion. Also they contain vitamin A, B, C and K (essential in many blood clotting factors). Rich in antioxidants and flavonoids.

Cantaloupe: Rich in vitamins and minerals, their intake helps to prevent blood clots. It has mild laxative effects, diuretic and antirheumatic facilitate digestion and colon cleansing.

Moral: One of the main advantages that can help the morale is by their fruits, as their consumption has laxative effects (constipation, irritable bowel syndrome) and are rich in fiber.

Banana: Besides having good amounts of potassium and other vitamins. In the case of not being intolerant banana it helps protect the stomach mucous membrane, preventing and healing ulcers and facilitate digestion. Its mild diuretic effect regulates body fluids and is also a good source of energy. Remember that the lower maturation process will lower its glycemic index (slower release of glucose in the blood).

Barley: We can also consume other grains such as corn, wheat or rye. Rich in vitamins and minerals (also contains eight essential amino acids therefore are attributed great benefits). Here we focus on your digestive support as it has been traditionally used to treat diarrhea, slow digestion, arteriosclerosis and diabetes.

Tamarind: It is rich in citric, tartaric and malic acids. Purifying the stomach and liver, so its consumption is highly digestive and very mild laxative. Its pulp is rich in thiamine (vitamin B1), used for the proper functioning of the nervous, digestive and muscular system so it is a great fi toni sing besides exercise that could prevent arteriosclerosis.

Cabbage: Has a high content of glutamine, vitamin C (more than oranges) and calcium (more than milk). Along with broccoli, or fl coli or cabbage could prevent many cancers as it is rich in alpha-linoliecos acid (omega 3). It is highly digestive, (to treat stomach ulcers and duodenum). Diuretic and antiin amatoria fl (deflating loving arteries and the heart muscle).

Tarragon or "Dragoncillo" There are scientific studies regarding the effectiveness of tarragon in the treatment of disorders digestive and as an appetite stimulant. also helps digest fats, encouraging the formation of gastric juices and bile increasing activity. This process can facilitate digestion eliminating toxins. Tarragon infusion can combat intestinal worms fresh leaves can also be chewed for toothache because it has analgesic and anti-in flammatory properties.

Milk Thistle: This plant could be gold natural liver protectors. This is because containing silymarin substance that detoxifies the liver and gall bladder (cirrhosis, hepatitis, fatty liver ...) reducing the damage caused by certain drugs such as antivirals, analgesics, antibiotics and antiinflammatory. Intervenes in cases of urolithiasis (kidney stones and gall bladder). Regulates cholesterol levels and blood glucose, relieving the pancreas release insulin. It also promotes the death of many cells that might be cancerous, this is also because it prevents lipid peroxidation (antioxidant action in fat tissues).

Fumaria: Very digestive medicinal plant and is also widely used as a liver protector. Would combat intestinal parasites and stomach discomfort. By its antimicrobial action can be used as topical to skin conditions such as acne, boils, sores, ulcers, urticaria or jaundice.

Radish: Along with garlic and onions they contain volatile sulfur components that could prevent many types of cancer. Digestive, bowel function support against ulcers and gastritis. Diuretic and rich in vitamin C.

Loosestrife (Arroyuella or puffin): very astringent, laxative and anti-in fl amatory plant. Interesting in cases of inflammation, bowel irritation and diseases of the colon. Antidiarreica also thanks to the pectin and tannins. Externally it used as eye drops and for skin conditions (eczema, herpes, etc.).

Goldenseal (Hydrastis canadensis): This herb is bactericidal, antiseptic and antiin fl ammatory circulatory (varices, hemorrhoids and hematomas). Highly digestible. Promotes the proper functioning of the pancreas and liver. Fights urinary tract infections and stomach. You can improve diabetes, this is because one of its alkaloids (berberine) regulates blood glucose and improves digestion. Outwardly it used for small wounds, mouthwash and sore throat. Also as eye drops and eyelid inflammation. It can support as a complement to preventive malaria when traveling because it promotes liver function. Continue studying the benefits of this herb as

It has many properties similar to ginseng and consult a specialist.

Cassia or "Chinese Canela" (Cinnamomum cassia): This plant belongs to the same family as cinnamon, functioning as a natural antiseptic, reducing diarrhea and stomach ailments besides being very digestible. Also it has other properties when added to the infusion as astringent, analgesic and soothing cramps and nausea. It can be obtained as an oil and applied to the skin on the areas in loved fl.

Oregano: Rich in beta-cario lina fi (substance antiin amatoria fl), antioxidants, polyphenols and vitamin E. Highly digestive oregano combat parasites and various urinaras infections. This is due to its antibiotic and antimicrobial properties. It also helps the liver function. As an infusion also has benefits expectorant and carminative (outgassing of the digestive tract).
Besides the ocean it has enormous amounts of calcium and potassium which can bene fi t the skeletal system.

Rosemary: Highly diuretic, carminative, digestive and expectorant. Packed with antioxidants plus fiber, potassium, iron and vitamin C. The consumption of rosemary infusion can alleviate many conditions and stomach problems as it is analgesic and antiviral improving blood flow, destroying microorganisms and stimulating bile secretion.

Cumin: Also with large amounts of calcium and potassium cumin it is a valuable ingredient as a diuretic, removing body fluids, as hypoglycemic, regulating the levels of blood glucose. And especially as a carminative and antispasmodic facilitating the expulsion of gases accumulated in the digestive tract and improving digestion. Galactógenas also has properties, ie, it could encourage the production of milk in nursing women.

Regarding the digestive system and the accumulated ammonia after exercise, in the market there are numerous elevators PH herbal that could help improve digestion, reduce acidity and alkalizing blood, recovering from a better shape after activity physical or workday. You can also choose lemon, rich in vitamin C, diuretic, antibacterial, antiseptic and toni fi cant (a major alkalizing there) and taken with warm water every morning, citric acid and ascorbic acid containing help eliminate acidity your body, relieving pain and fatigue, stimulating the immune system and facilitate digestion. As well as important resources can also get sodium bicarbonate or "salts fruit" as they are potent acid but use them with caution. Studies and possible evidence that intake of alkaline foods including lemon and adding a little baking soda (as applicable) may alleviate or prevent many cancer cells from spreading even to eliminate as many viruses and bacteria They die in an alkaline medium. Carefully document more about it and talk to your doctor and specialists.

The secret is "be" in order to have; you will not see abundance in your life until you do not see it first in your mind.

15. SUPPORT AND ACTIVE INGREDIENTS FOR JOINTS

Almost culminating this great second part of the book, what's next in this chapter are some plants and principles that can bene fi ciarle for moments of physical activity, relieving joint fatigue of everyday life or to know them and use them as professional health evaluation or help the treatment of conditions that may limit the ability to move.

Ginger: It appears again as external use to support in improving arthritis, osteoarthritis, or muscle aches, toothaches and deflating love joints.

Rosemary: His alcohol and oil is very interesting for rheumatism, arthritis pain, and those headaches of nervous origin. You can apply it in the joints before physical or evening for relaxation and decongestion activity.
Also as an infusion in water bath for muscle pain.

Eucalyptus: Its essential oil is interesting to infections genitourinary tract and to apply on muscles and joints relieving the physical fatigue.

Coriander: You can be obtained for use topically as a poultice for joint pain by its properties antiin fl ammatory and analgesic.

White Sauce: Its content splashes becomes the body salicylic acid which reduces the sensation of pain in the body. It can be applied externally to prevent infection and inflammation.

Oregano: External use oil can be applied to reduce pain and inflammation. It is also an ideal antiseptic bath water.

Harpago fi to: Its essential oil relieves arthritis, osteoarthritis, arthritis and other musculoskeletal conditions as it is antiin-inflammatory and analgesic (rich in iridoid glycosides, flavonoids, polyphenols and harpágidos).Alsoitusedforbumps and bruises.

Arnica Montana: Basis of many creams and components to treat pain, this species is very important for its various properties. Rich in flavonoids, mucilages and alkaloids than betaine and arnicina tonify allowing the circulatory system, moisturizing joints.

Hypericum: The application of the oil has astringent, antiin ammatory and healing skin fl and can also be bene fi cial if abrasions or burns.

Calendula: Used for deflating love and disinfect the area of application. It is very rich in antioxidants besides promote circulation.

Rosehip: Among its many properties you can use oil to moisturize your skin and relieve pain points. It can be applied on stretch marks, blemishes and wrinkles, aid healing, burns and improve conditions caused skin as it is rich in vitamin A, C, E and essential fatty acids.

In the market you can find also different essences, oils, creams or sprays herbal to apply the joint or muscle areas. Many use capsaicin (the active ingredient in hot peppers) as an active ingredient to give effect feels the heat or peppermint, turpentine, menthol or camphor to give that feeling cold. Always attend its purity, quality components and are a reliable source.

Do not ask permission to fulfill your dreams, valórate! not everyone understands art, remember that a diamond is cut under pressure. Use things that happen to you as inspiration!

16. HELP IN DEFICIENCY STATES AND GENERAL HEALTH PROBLEMS

In this final part you will find a number of plants that stand out much for its antibiotic properties (including medicinal principles), which are very interesting to bene fi ciarle in different conditions and strengthen your immune system in general. Take complete freedom to use this information as often as their sufficient.

Cat's claw (Uncaria tomentosa) Antioxidant and natural antibiotic. Its properties are used to kill certain bacteria and viruses. It is analgesic, antiseptic and anti-in fl ammatory so may favor certain conditions (arthritis, osteoarthritis, gout ...) and respiratory and urinary infections. Cat's claw also promotes improved circulation unblocking arteries and preventing thromboses and clots. In addition to regulating blood sugar, strengthens the immune system.

Echinacea: This native species of North America is also a potent natural antibiotic and could be used for colds, colds, flu and viral infections of the respiratory tract well.

Thyme: Antiparasitic, disinfectant, antimicrobial, anti-catarrhal, expectorant, muscle relaxant, digestive and healing. It can also be mixed with laurel since its leaves are antiseptic and expectorants (used as rinses in bucco-pharyngeal cases of infections or chronic bronchitis).

Eucalyptus: This plant also appears here because part used for joints and pain points as we saw in the previous chapter is a powerful disinfectant, decongestant and expectorant. Treats lung infections, colds, colds and sore throats. You can mix with incense or mint as it can reduce coughing, bronchitis and decongest the respiratory tract or ginger as it is antiin-inflammatory and analgesic, and other plants.

Sage: This plant considered a natural antibiotic. Used for respiratory conditions (chest throat) and to relieve colds. Externally mouthwash (gums, ulcers and teeth) and applied to the skin as healing for minor cuts or infections. It is rich in zinc and in particular is taken into tea by upper gastrointestinal relieving properties gastritis, diarrhea, ulcers, nerves and other stomach problems. Taken after meals may reduce blood glucose. If women are not recommended for use during pregnancy because this plant contains thujone and different ellagic and oleanolic that could cause birth acids. It can also be added to bath water as a muscle relaxant.

Filipendula Ulmaria: One of the main properties of this plant is that it is very rich in silicates salicylic acid and so has been used for fever and flu states for its analgesic, antibiotic antiin ammatory and fl. You can contribute to the relief of headache, joint and some urinary tract infections.

Eufrasia: Used especially for eye diseases (conjunctivitis, inflammation of the eyelids, sties, eyestrain) and respiratory (stomatitis, rhinitis, defamation of the mucosa of the nasal passages, throat, colds and flu). It is also highly digestive for its flavonoid content (quercetósidos), glycosides, phenolic acids, tannins and lignans that make antiin amatoria, antiseptic and healing fl.

Plantain (Plantago major): It is antibacterial, astringent, antiseptic, antiin amatory, expectorant diuretic plus fl. Plant for treating colds, bronchitis and asthma plus some UTIs In gargle used can relieve angina and as eye drops is indicated for conjunctivitis and inflammation of the eyelids. It is also highly digestible and can be applied to the skin for small wounds, in fl ammation, cuts and bites.

Myrrh: For its richness in antioxidants this plant can be used to treat gingivitis and mouth sores. An oil can also be applied in fl mild skin inflammations, abrasions, acne or rash.

Or black poplar elm (Ulmus carpinifolia): It contains Salicia and may have benefits as well as anti-in fl amatory antiseptic, digestive and expectorant. (It has been used to improve some treatments on the respiratory tract). And analgesic properties depending on symptoms can help reduce fever.

Pelargonium (Pelargonium sidoides): This medicinal native South area can help in cases of bronchitis, tonsillitis, pharyngitis, sinusitis and various viral respiratory tract infections. Its antibacterial and antiviral actions stimulate the production of phagocytes, immune function keys.

Cat foot (Antennaria dioica): This species contains abundant mucilage, flavonoids and potassium salts (very diuretic). may be indicated for respiratory diseases such as bronchitis and if pharyngitis, stomach or gastritis as cholecystitis, and bladder such as cystitis and oliguria.

Pine (Pinus sylvestris) Leaves and bark are rich in many properties such as turpentine, tannin, various acids such as ascorbic acid (vitamin C), carotenoids, flavonoids, lutein and quercetin. Its essential oil has expectorant properties,

Balsamic and antiseptic that which could favor in respiratory symptoms. It is also antiin-inflammatory and diuretic which has been used in drop boxes, gallstones, cystitis and oliguria (infection and inflammation of the bladder and decreasing the normal volume of urine respectively).

Licorice (Glycyrrhiza glabra): This herb is rich in one of its natural components, glycyrrhizin. It is antispasmodic, anti-in fl amatory and antacid so it can be ideal for reducing heartburn, indigestion and deflating the gastric mucosa love. Also it exerts a protective function of the liver (as in cases of hepatitis, cirrhosis or liver decongestion) and airway (sore throat, cough, colds and bronchitis).

Elderberry, elderberry flower (Sambucus nigra): It hosts a lot of properties that could help fight many respiratory conditions and also is antiviral and bactericidal antiinflamatory. The flowers in favor elderberry colds and flu-like processes. It can be mixed with lemon balm, eucalyptus, rosemary, thyme and especially with mint. Very diuretic, used to relieve fluid retention and uric acid, while improving urinary and kidney infections (inflammation, calculations ...). Its berries are also edible but monitor the state of maturation, since the leaves, bark and fruit can harbor immaturity in certain toxicity. Check with your specialist.

Vanilla (Vanilla planifolia): Besides being used as a spice that brings a fresh, deep and aromatic taste in many culinary preparations, also it contains many medicinal properties as it is a tranquilizer and natural antibiotic. In fact it is the only edible orchid. It contains salicylic acid making it very analgesic (for muscle pains and stomach). It reduces fever since it is abundant in benzoic acid and eugenol (fever-reducing components). And also it supports digestion (contains catechins), stimulates the production of bile and is rich in antioxidants.

Verbena (Verbena officinalis of): The active ingredients of this plant (iridoid glycosides, phenylpropanoids, and caffeic ursóalico) make it stand out as an analgesic and natural antibiotic. Externally it used against all kinds of joint pain and internally as antispasmodic and febrifuge (colds, respiratory infections, cough, bronchitis) as well as being toni fi cant and digestive.

Kombucha: This native of China and extended in several countries and probiotic drink is made with fermented black tea to which are added certain sugars to feed the bacteria and fungi diversity are also added. The most common genera that can be found in this drink or tea are kombuchae Gluconacetobacter, Acetobacter, lactobacillus,

Pediococcus and kombuchaensis Zygosaccharomyces. These organisms enter the body providing numerous bene fi ts helping improve intestinal digestion. Rich in vitamin C and B, amino acids and enzymes. Currently already commercially it produced for many supermarkets and specialty stores. Ables ask fi sources and attend review its quality seals.

After reading about all these genres also be re-destacarle as benefit immune wealth of vitamin C in certain foods, very important for the body in different vital functions (one iron absorption). For example remember that you have the orange or the lemon, loaded with anti-oxidants, may reduce hypertension, heartburn, besides being diuretics (ulcers, gout, arthritis, atherosclerosis, constipation) and anticancer antiseptics. You can also find the Red pepper after Australian kakadu (5 g. of vitamin C per 100 g.), the camucamu (Myrciaria dubia) South American (3 g. per 100 g.), acerola, blackcurrants and parsley, pepper is one of the genres that contain more vitamin C, even surpassing citrus. Very important to prevent colds and favor the digestive system (stomach ulcers, heartburn). It contains next to tomatoes, lycopene, one of the best antioxidants responsible for decontaminating the body of free radicals. It is also abundant in tryptophan and vitamin A. Note also that acerola (Malpighia emarginata), after Australian kakadu and Camu Camu is possibly one of the fruits with more vitamin C in the world studied and even sold in capsules or tablets as food supplement (about 2 grams of vitamin C per 100 g. compared with 50 mg of an orange), shaping it as a potent antioxidant slowing the causes of oxidative stress that can damage cells.

Remember that things do not happen to you to give up or break you are to break and rebuild you again, harder, smarter, more experienced and determination. Why fear progress and what makes you getting stronger? Things do not happen "for you" happen "to you", not "everything happens me me" is "teaching me life," he discovers the teaching behind every situation and do different things, that alone will be one step far ahead of most.

17. WE REACH THE END, AND NOW WHAT?

And now that? What should you do? Where do you start? I always say, talk is easy, it is very important to know how much but still is more how you apply.

I hope you enjoyed reading this book as I have done writing. I am totally convinced of it. Fully I trust you to use in the best way possible the principles I have mentioned in this book to dramatically improve your life.

In my experience, the mere fact that you read, you will not bring any result. There is no difference between who can not read and do not apply what you read. For this reason and as in any other area of your life, reading is a start, but if you want success out there, all we will have are your actions. In the first part of this book (Chapter 1 through 6) I have given you numerous supplements and nutritional principles to complement your meal plan, physical activity and rest. I encourage you to reread all the sections as often as their fi cient as you obtain information more about it.

In the second part (Chapters 7 to 16) have learned the advantages and benefits of knowing and classify according to the condition, symptom, prevention or momentum of improvement, many medicinal plants and genres in order to help you improve your fitness, wellness and lifestyle. Since many drinks "detox", teas, anabolic plants, revitalizing, digestive, diuretic ... and countless species in your power to make life much better.

That's why I suggest that because improve your condition invite you to reread this book from beginning to end at least once a month during the following years (including reflections to give you strength and I do not consider knowledge without action and motivation without attitude). Maybe you tell me: << What do I need to do if I already I read >>?. Very good question but there is an equally good answer: repetition, consistency and discipline are accompanied by the attitude of learning mothers. Therefore, the more you study this book you will quickly integrate into you all concepts. Believe me, there is no greater investment, more profitable and more fruitful than you can do yourself.

Be sure to visit me in my social networks or officers to hear from you and how much I could help this book. Your opinion interests me and in fact if you have any questions, suggestions or need my support or guide can also write. I'll be happy to read you. I also still learning my way to success daily and if you already know me, but my life are business, education financial and
self-improvement, the area of health and fitness is no less important to me. What better way then that helping others achieve their own goals! My purpose is to inspire and motivate millions of people to be its best through financial education, achievement of objectives, goals and daily strategies (or in this case, physical health) so that they can thus achieve excellence and personal welfare. So all areas are important: mental, emotional, spiritual, physical ... and are extremely linked. Neglecting health would make life lacked any sense.

I feel really fortunate to create books, teach courses, podcasts, interviews, media appearances, contributions on digital platforms in addition to various business campaign services such as consulting, techniques and strategies to transform and improve the lives of people on a permanent basis. Heart I invite you to continue learning in our social networks and in various sources and means for you to follow training and can be better informed to make better future decisions. Remember that you can write us for any project, query or suggestion to the following email:

<u>clientes@valentinlopez.org</u>

That's all for now. Totally grateful for spend your valuable time reading this book. Thanks from me and on behalf of the entire team. Best wishes and I hope to meet you in person soon.

Your attitude defines your altitude,

Valentín López

18. BIBLIOGRAPHY

Bean, Anita, *The Complete Guide to Nutrition athlete,* Paidotribo.

Benardot, Dan, *Advanced Sports Nutrition,* Tutor.

Williams, Melvin H., *Nutrition for health, fitness and sports,* Old Dominion University, Paidotribo.

Haff, Gregory G. and Triplett, N. Travis, *Early strength training and fitness NCSA,* Paidotribo.

Ratamess, Nicholas, *ACSM Manual of strength training and fitness,* American College of Sports Medicine, Paidotribo.

Clark, Nancy, *Sports nutrition guide Nancy Clark,* Paidotribo.

Hernandez, Angel G., *Treaty Nutrition,* Panamericana.

Whitney, Eleanor N., *General Nutrition Treaty,* Paidotribo.

Verdu, Jose M., *Nutrition and Food, Nutrients and Food; fi physiological and pathological situations,* Ergon.

Ross, Catharine A., *Nutrition in Health and Disease,* Wolters Kluwer Health, Lippincott Williams and Wilkins.

Roman, Daniel A., *Diet therapy, Clinical Nutrition and Metabolism,* Diaz de Santos.

Erdman, John W., *Nutrition and diet in disease prevention,* McGraw-Hill.

Stipanuk, and Martha H. Caudill, Marie A., *Biochemical, Physiological, and Molecular Aspects of Human Nutrition,* Elsevier Science.

Roldán, Alfredo A., *Guide to natural remedies and dietary supplements star,* Arcopress.

Vanaclocha, Bernat and Cañigueral, Salvador, Phytotherapy: *Vademecum prescription,* Elsevier Masson.

Berdonces, Jose L., *Great Dictionary of medicinal plants, description and applications: The most comprehensive book on Phytotherapy,* Ambarocean.

Garcia, C. and Solis Encarna, Isabel M., *Phytotherapy manual,* Elsevier Spain.

Has Palazuelos, Francisco J., *Practical use of Phytotherapy in gynecology,* Panamericana.

Molto Ripoll, Juan Pablo and Garrido C., Josep, *Traditional Chinese herbal medicine with Western plants; the most important plants in the West for Traditional Chinese Medicine,* Dilemma.

Kuklinski, Claudia, *Farmaconogsia; studies of drugs and medicinal substances of natural origin,* Omega.

Bruneton, Jean, *Farmaconogsia, Phytochemistry, medicinal plants,* Acribia.

Mahan, and Kathleen L. Raymond, Janice L., *Krause's Food & Nutrition care process,* Saunders.

Poindexter, Brenda and Karpen, Heidi, *Current Concepts in Neonatal Nutrition,* Elsevier.

Wémeau, JL, JL and Vialettes B. Schlienger, *Endocrinologie, Diabète, métabolisme et Nutrition,* Elsevier Masson.

Roth, Sara L. and Schlenker, Eleanor, *Williams' Essentials of Nutrition and Diet Therapy,* Mosby.

Morley, John E., *Nutrition in Older Adults; Geriatric Medicine Clinics in,* Elsevier.

Foster, J., Smith, M. and Riby, L., *Nutrition and Mental Performance: A Lifespan Perspective,* Macmillan Childrens.

Walkingshaw, Bonnie C., *R. Long, Sara and Grodner, Michele, Foundations and Clinical Applications Nutritional,* Mosby.

Mills, Simon and Bone, Kerry, *Principles and Practice of Phytotherapy,* Churchill Livingstone.

Gibbons, Simon Barnes, Joanne and Heinrich, Michael, *Fundamentals of Pharmacognosy and Phytotherapy,* Churchill Livingstone.

Ferriss, Timothy, *Titans weapons,* Deusto.

Raubenheimer, David and Simpson, Stephen J., *The Nature of Nutrition,* Princeton University Press.

My total gratitude to the authors cited bibliographic cos as they have been a great reference for me. Thanks to all of them for their great works and which certainly have exerted an enormous influence in my life and in the creation of this book. Also thank all the entrepreneurs and personalities who have contributed to this book. In addition to family and friends. We have certainly built something great.